108 Pearls

to Awaken Your
Healing Potential

ALSO BY MIMI GUARNERI, M.D.

The Heart Speaks: A Cardiologist Reveals the Secret Language of Healing

•••

HAY HOUSE TITLES OF RELATED INTEREST

YOU CAN HEAL YOUR LIFE, the movie, starring Louise Hay & Friends
(available as a 1-DVD program and an expanded 2-DVD set)
Watch the trailer at: www.LouiseHayMovie.com

THE SHIFT, the movie,
starring Dr. Wayne W. Dyer
(available as a 1-DVD program and an expanded 2-DVD set)
Watch the trailer at: www.DyerMovie.com

•••

*HEAL YOUR MIND: Your Prescription for Wholeness through Medicine,
Affirmations, and Intuition,* by Mona Lisa Schulz M.D., Ph.D.,
and Louise Hay

LOVING YOURSELF TO GREAT HEALTH: Thoughts & Food—the Ultimate Diet,
by Louise Hay, Ahlea Khadro, and Heather Dane

*MEDICAL MEDIUM: Secrets Behind Chronic and Mystery Illness and How to
Finally Heal,* by Anthony William

YOU ARE THE PLACEBO: Making Your Mind Matter, by Dr. Joe Dispenza

Please visit:

Mimi Guarneri: www.mimiguarnerimd.com
Hay House USA: www.hayhouse.com®
Hay House Australia: www.hayhouse.com.au
Hay House UK: www.hayhouse.co.uk
Hay House South Africa: www.hayhouse.co.za
Hay House India: www.hayhouse.co.in

108 Pearls

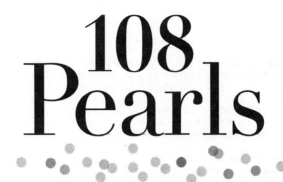

to Awaken Your Healing Potential

Mimi Guarneri, M.D.

HAY HOUSE, INC.
Carlsbad, California • New York City
London • Sydney • Johannesburg
Vancouver • New Delhi

Copyright © 2017 by Mimi Guarneri, M.D.

Published and distributed in the United States by: Hay House, Inc.: www.hay house.com® • *Published and distributed in Australia by:* Hay House Australia Pty. Ltd.: www.hayhouse.com.au • *Published and distributed in the United Kingdom by:* Hay House UK, Ltd.: www.hayhouse.co.uk • *Published and distributed in the Republic of South Africa by:* Hay House SA (Pty), Ltd.: www.hayhouse.co.za • *Distributed in Canada by:* Raincoast Books: www.raincoast.com • *Published in India by:* Hay House Publishers India: www.hayhouse.co.in

Editors: Jeanne Bellezzo, writeideas.biz; and Gail Rose, anantacreativegroup.com
Cover design: Karla Baker • *Interior design:* Bryn Starr Best

**Cataloging-in-Publication Data
is on file with the Library of Congress**

ISBN: 978-1-4019-4577-0

10 9 8 7 6 5 4 3
1st edition, April 2017

Printed in the United States of America

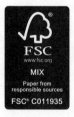
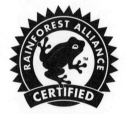

To my patients, who have taught me the power of the human spirit.

*To my friends and colleagues, Mitch Gaynor and Lee Lipsenthal,
who in their short lives strengthened me with their wisdom and love.*

*To my brother, Dominick, and my cousin, John, who taught
me to celebrate each and every day of this human life.*

*To Rauni Prittinen King, my friend, colleague, and co-visionary
in creating a health care system that is the
essence of science and compassion.*

*And to all my colleagues who are courageous enough to
stand strong and deliver care focused on health creation
for humanity and the planet.*

CONTENTS

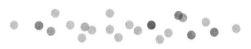

FOREWORD

For many years, Mimi Guarneri has traveled to some of the most remote and impoverished areas of the world to help those in critical need of health-care services. Her noble work goes beyond the finite number of lives she saves and heals on each mission. Their health is our health. Their behaviors and survival methods have a profound effect on the overall health of our planet, just as our own habits do. We are one world.

As you start your own step-by-step journey to optimal health, remember that human health is intimately connected to the health of the planet, which is in rapid and serious decline. For 40 years, I have been one of many voices warning society about the impending environmental crisis threatening our world. We are now at a crossroads concerning environmental issues in general, and climate change in particular.

This is not an issue we can continue to ignore or dismiss. We are running out of time. Our planet is in need of healing now.

Air pollution levels are at an all-time high and getting worse. Over the past few decades, our ecosystem has been speaking out in a number of ways: record hot temperatures, devastating hurricanes and typhoons, major droughts, unprecedented snowfalls, and more. The summer Arctic Sea ice pack has decreased by more than 30 percent since the 1980s. Records tell us that average temperatures worldwide are rising; if this trend continues, by midcentury, no ecosystem in known history will ever have seen such a warm planet. We are heading into uncharted territory.

The record drought in California in recent years and its adverse impact on the state, one of the most technologically advanced regions of the world, is a stark reminder that everyone, not just the poor or the poor nations, is vulnerable to drastic climate changes.

There has long been talk about addressing the problem, but little has been done in the way of action. We have delayed taking significant action for so long that if we don't do something in the next few years—not the next 50 years or the next 10 years, but the next few years—we will be pushing the ecosystem to extremes it has never seen.

What needs to happen before we as a society wake up and decide that enough is enough? Part of the problem is that we believe the air we breathe belongs to everyone. If the air in our homes were polluted, we would call someone out to fix it. But when the air on our planet is polluted, we expect someone else to take care of it.

When the planet gets too hot, the privileged among us can protect ourselves with more air-conditioning. However, there are three billion poor people in the world who are living in tropical countries with no access to indoor climate control. When the sea level rises so high that we lose entire islands, we can build homes high on a mountain. We will lose some money but not our lives. Yet many others are one hurricane or one drought away from extinction.

It is a moral and ethical issue on many dimensions. We inherited a beautiful planet. When we die, we will be handing the next generation a damaged planet with extreme air pollution, contaminated oceans, devastated rain forests, mountains without snowpacks or glaciers, and entire species that have disappeared. Generations to come will be adversely affected, since the carbon pollution from fossil fuels and the resulting climate changes can last for more than 1,000 years. They will wonder why we ignored compelling scientific evidence and advice to mitigate. The costs of mitigating the changes are so low compared with the damages that they will find it impossible to think of us, their ancestors, as "intelligent life"!

It is up to us to decide: Do we hand the planet to the next generation without a scratch? Or do we continue to exploit it as much as possible and hope they are smart enough to figure it out?

Solutions to these problems exist, but they require the rest of us to fundamentally change our attitudes toward nature and toward each other and to strive to work for the common good. For instance, there are three billion people who are forced by poverty to cook with dung, wood, and crop wastes. These fires are not only a major source of soot but also the cause of death of three million people annually—mostly women and infants. I have started Project Surya (www.projectsurya.org), which has documented the climate and health effects of the soot from cooking and identified a stove that reduces the soot drastically. The stoves cost about $70 each—pocket change for many of us, but close to six weeks of take-home pay for these people.

So how can we as individuals make a difference as part of our own paths to health and healing?

We can become informed, educated citizens, and we can pass our education on at every opportunity. We can organize to protect the planet. We can sponsor charitable events to raise awareness of the environment. We can take real steps to reduce our energy consumption, such as with the food we eat and the gas we put in our cars. Ideally, along with cutting back our energy use, we could potentially convert all our energy sources to renewable fuels.

Did you know that the emissions from the gallons of fuel you put in your gas tank stay in the air for hundreds, even thousands, of years? Did you know that wasted food is the third-largest source of global warming pollution? Rotting food produces methane, a natural gas, which remains in the environment for 15 years and is the second-largest contributor to climate change. Yet one-third of the food we produce in the United States is wasted. From the grocery store to our own kitchen counter when the produce in the bins start to turn brown, we throw them away. Furthermore, meat production is highly energy intensive. And because the digestive system of cows is so inefficient, they are constantly emitting methane gas into the air.

There are small changes that we can make every day. We can take shorter showers and turn off the tap when we brush our teeth. We can buy food produced locally, which cuts down on the costs and emissions of trucking food across the country. We can adopt a vegan or vegetarian diet or simply eat less meat. Many across the country have pledged to have a meatless meal once or twice a week.

Remember, in protecting the earth, we also protect our children, our grandchildren, and *their* children. After all, we do our best to leave behind a nice home for our children. Shouldn't we try just as hard to leave behind a habitable planet to build that home?

When it comes to healing the planet, the first steps must take place within each individual person. You can start today by taking control of your own health with the 108 pearls of wisdom that Dr. Guarneri guides you through so beautifully in this book. Know that when you walk or bike to work, you are doing as much for the health of the planet as you are for your own. When you reduce the meat in your diet or shop at local markets, you are reducing your carbon footprint. When you stop using plastic water bottles, you are reducing the size of landfills as well as your exposure to chemicals. This list goes on. There isn't a suggestion in this book that doesn't help fulfill a dream for a healthier planet.

"What is personal is truly universal," says Dr. Guarneri. Take her words to heart as you begin your journey.

— Dr. Veerabhadran Ramanathan

Dr. Veerabhadran Ramanathan is a distinguished professor of atmospheric and climate sciences at the Scripps Institution of Oceanography at the University of California, San Diego, and UNESCO Professor of Climate and Policy, TERI University, Delhi. A member of the Intergovernmental Panel on Climate Change (IPCC), a United Nations body awarded the Nobel Prize in 2007, he was honored as the 2013 Champion of Earth for Science and Innovation by the United Nations and named as the 2014 Global Thinker by Foreign Policy magazine. He was recently honored as a council member of Pope Francis's Pontifical Academy of Sciences. In this capacity, he has briefed the pope on sustainability and climate change and is co-organizing a climate change summit at the Vatican chaired by UN Secretary-General Ban Ki-moon.

INTRODUCTION

What if you woke up one morning and were living the life you always imagined? What would that look like? Better yet, what would that feel like? Would you have an abundance of material things or an endless supply of energy? Would you be surrounded by unlimited wealth or a few close friends and family? It's almost impossible to picture an ideal life void of good health and loving relationships.

Creating and preserving our health should be one of the primary goals in life. After all, without our health we are unable to achieve our full potential as human beings. I define *optimal health* as the conscious pursuit of the highest level of functioning an individual can achieve. It includes a healthy balance of the physical, mental, emotional, spiritual, environmental, and social aspects of being human. For some people, optimal health might mean being able to climb Mount Everest. For others, it might mean being able to shop, cook, and care for their own homes.

As a physician, I hear patients say over and over, "I would gladly give up my wealth just to have back my health."

How do we preserve our health in a world filled with demands, conflicting information, and suffering? The answer is simple: we take steps—maybe just one at a time—and begin a lifelong journey of transformation. We ask questions. We get educated. We learn about nutrition and supplements. We explore our spirituality. With each step we take, we put knowledge into practice until our lives are deeply transformed.

Let's start by taking a deep breath and filling our hearts with loving-kindness—for ourselves, our loved ones, and our planet. If you have ever practiced yoga, centering prayer, or guided meditation, your instructor may have asked you to recite a sacred word or chant to release you from your busy day and bring you into the present moment. This is where transformation begins.

I like to pray using a strand of *mala* beads. Malas are strings of 108 beads used to count during mantra meditations. Mine are made of pearl, a strong and beautiful gemstone with mysterious healing powers that reminds me that beauty lies within every new challenge. The pearl is created out of pain and suffering. As an irritating grain of sand settles in the oyster, the oyster responds by creating layers and layers of a healing salve. The end result is a pearl. The pearl is a metaphor for life.

As I feel the smooth perfection of each pearl's surface beneath my fingers, I begin to chant and drift into a transformative state of calm resolve. With each breath I take, I can feel life's vital force flowing through every cell in my body.

Global healing traditions such as Ayurveda and Traditional Chinese Medicine teach us that there are seven major chakras or energy centers in the body, and each is associated with a physical, emotional, or mental function. When the flow of energy in one or more of these regions becomes blocked, illness related to that energy center may result. When our chakras are open, there is a healthy flow of energy throughout our body that is healing and restorative.

It is not surprising that the fourth chakra—the heart chakra—is my favorite. It is where love, compassion, and forgiveness reside.

As a cardiologist, I am taught to save lives by opening blocked arteries with metal sleeves called stents. Stents scaffold the artery open and restore the healthy flow of blood to the heart. It is both a mechanical procedure and a true miracle of modern medicine, one that I have performed thousands of times during my career.

Yet another kind of heart opening occurs when we let love, compassion, and purpose guide our choices: when we honor our bodies and respect the planet, give our time to friends and loved ones, engage in meaningful work and community activities, and remain true to our deepest beliefs and values.

This is the foundation of optimal health, which we as physicians are privileged to support with advanced medical technology as well as the wisdom of all global healing traditions. I believe there are many paths to health and healing, and they all begin in our hearts—with the desire to live the kind of lives that not only sustain us but also awaken our spirits, energize our minds, and nourish our bodies.

Within these pages, I have developed a comprehensive, step-by-step program that addresses everything from the foods you eat to the relationships you cultivate, to the way you work and play, to the amount of stress in your life and how you can transform it. Each step holds a new pearl of knowledge, another opening to the greater path of healing. Take each of these 108 pearls to heart.

Let's Start at 108. And Take the First Step.

Why 108 pearls? As I mentioned, there are 108 beads on a traditional mala, which is used for counting or chanting a mantra or sacred word, much like a string of rosary beads used by Catholics in prayer. The number 108 is considered to be sacred in Hinduism, where repetitive prayer is embedded into the everyday experience (which, of course, is true in most every culture).

As a young girl, I was taught to pray the rosary, but I did not understand the power behind this simple technique. It was years later, during a trip to India, that I learned to chant a simple mantra on a mala, which felt right at home in my hands. Holding the mala and reciting the mantra helped me to focus my mind and let go of worry. By the time I reached 108, I felt revived, focused, and, most important, at peace.

The steps in this program are designed to prevent and improve common diseases utilizing the science of health. Throughout the process, you will be asked to visualize your healthiest, happiest, and most prosperous self. You will be given the knowledge, the tools, and the support you need to get there. Set your intention on the life you always imagined. How does it look? How does it feel?

Treating disease after it occurs is not the solution. Macro- and micronutrition, supplements, stress management, enhanced resiliency, and spirituality are just a few of the key components to health and longevity. These pearls will teach you everything you need to know to stay healthy from a mind-body-spirit perspective. Each step is a simple solution that you can put into practice, often immediately.

Remember, the steps provide information that leads to knowledge, but putting each step to practice in your life is what leads to transformation. Don't rush to complete them all at once. Some will be easy for you; others are more challenging. I recommend reading each step and considering how you might apply it in your daily life before moving on to the next. Before you know it, you will have 108 pearls of wisdom empowering your journey to health and healing.

• ● •

CHAPTER 1

Establish Your Foundation for Health

As you begin your journey of health creation, you will be invited to take simple yet powerful steps to heal, strengthen, and transform your life. I recommend that you start by setting aside some time to answer a few questions and find out some information about yourself that sets your foundation of health.

1. Evaluate Your Overall Health.

Before you read further in the book, write out your answers to the following questions. Evaluate yourself again after you complete the program, and compare your answers from before and after.

- **How would you describe your physical health?** Do you feel well and have enough energy to get through the day? Do you take medications to treat physical challenges such as diabetes or high blood pressure? Is there something you would like to do but can't because it's too physically demanding? How might your health be better?

- **How would you describe your mental or emotional health?** Do you have anxiety or depression? Would you describe your life as stressful? Are you happy and content? Are you optimistic? Are you irritable and angry?

- **Do you need medications or supplements to sleep?**
- **Do you feel socially connected and supported?** How is your relationship with your partner? Is it loving or do you "walk on eggshells" to keep the peace?
- **Do you feel a spiritual connection to something greater than yourself?**
- **What is your purpose in life?** What is your passion? What inspires you most?
- **Did you grow up in an emotionally challenging environment?** Were you close to your parents or caregivers? Did you have a warm relationship with them?
- **How do you relate to your physical environment?** Are you in touch with what is happening in the world around you?
- **Do you feel connected to nature?** Does being near water, mountains, fields, or woods affect your mood?

2. Know Your Cholesterol Numbers.

Not all cholesterol is bad. Without it, our bodies wouldn't be able to keep our cells healthy or produce important hormones such as estrogen and testosterone.

Cholesterol is a waxy substance found in the fats in our blood. Our liver manufactures all the cholesterol we need, but sometimes it makes too much in response to toxins such as mercury and other heavy metals. The modification of cholesterol can lead to blockages in your arteries and can increase your risk of heart disease and stroke.

While some people have genetic disorders that lead to high cholesterol, the condition is usually a result of lifestyle, hormones, and toxin exposure. What we eat and drink, how much alcohol we consume, how often we exercise, and even how stressed out we feel all contribute to our cholesterol levels.

After about age 40, most people should get a standard blood test called a lipid panel. The American College of Cardiology has specific guidelines for health-care providers to follow. If you have a family history of high cholesterol or heart disease, your physician may recommend checking your lipids more often or at a younger age.

A basic lipid panel report includes four important numbers: total cholesterol, HDL cholesterol, LDL cholesterol, and triglycerides.

- Total cholesterol is calculated by adding your HDL, LDL, and 20 percent of your triglyceride values.

- HDL stands for high-density lipoprotein. It is considered the "good" cholesterol. (My patients have taught me that the *H* in HDL is for the "happy" cholesterol.) There are several subtypes of HDL, most importantly HDL2B, which is the HDL responsible for pulling plaque out of our arteries.

- LDL stands for low-density lipoprotein. (My patients call this the "lousy" cholesterol.) It's common to hear that LDL causes plaque in the arteries, but this is not totally accurate. It is the type of LDL that is important. LDL comes in various sizes. Small particles are more aggressive and more likely to cause disease. LDL that is damaged, such as oxidized LDL, is more damaging to your arteries than large, fluffy LDL.

- Triglycerides are the main form of fat stored in our body. In fact, triglycerides fight with our good HDL cholesterol for space in our blood. As triglycerides go up, HDL goes down, and vice versa. If we can lower our triglycerides, we raise our good HDL.

However, the numbers you get in a basic lipid panel are just that—basic. I recommend asking your health-care provider for an advanced lipid panel, which includes LDL size and particle number and HDL2b levels. Make sure you also check your oxidized LDL, which is an important marker for inflammation. An additional important test is the measurement of apolipoprotein B (apo B), which is a measure of all the potential artery-clogging particles.

I set the following goals for my patients, especially those with vascular disease or diabetes, using my rule of the three 6s:

> *APO B—60 mg/dl*
> *HDL > 60 mg/dl*
> *LDL—60 to 70 mg/dl*

Oxidized LDL (OxLDL) should be under 45 mg/dl. Furthermore, your LDL particle number (the biggest predictor of vascular disease progression) should be less than 700 mg/dl. Triglycerides, the form of fat that comes from sugar and carbohydrates, should be less than 100 mg/dl.

3. Check Your Inflammation Levels.

Think about the last time you had a cut that became infected or the last time you had an allergic reaction. Your skin probably swelled and became red and tender. Swelling, redness, pain, immobility, and warmth are classic signs of inflammation. It is the body's natural response to an injury, infection, stress, foreign substances, or anything else that threatens our well-being. It is a crucial protective reaction that allows us to heal.

Acute inflammation usually lasts for days or, rarely, a few weeks. Bronchitis and tonsillitis are both examples of acute inflammation. (The suffix *-itis* means "inflammation.") Chronic inflammation, on the other hand, is like a smoldering fire. You may not even realize it is present, yet it can do an enormous amount of damage over the course of weeks, months, or even years. This is why your inflammatory markers are equally as important to know as your cholesterol numbers.

Any pain or swelling has associated inflammation. Your eyes water? Your joints ache? Your skin breaks out in a rash? These are signs of inflammation in your body—and where's there's smoke, there's probably fire.

Researchers are finding that chronic inflammation plays a significant role in serious diseases such as cancer, Alzheimer's disease, diabetes, and arthritis. Cardiologists now believe that inflammation is a bigger factor in coronary artery disease than is cholesterol. There are hundreds of autoimmune diseases, and every one of them is linked to inflammation.

There are simple blood tests that can help your health-care provider determine if you have inflammation. Some tests are specific for artery inflammation, such as the LpPLA2 and MPO (myeloperoxidase) tests, while others are less specific, such as the hs-CRP or high-sensitivity CRP test. Hs-CRP will tell us that inflammation is present in the body, but it is not specific as to where. For example, hs-CRP may be high from skin rashes such as psoriasis or arthritis, while LpPLA2 is more specific for inflammation in arteries.

I use a simple symptom questionnaire in my practice (see Appendix A). You can use it to uncover inflammation in all areas of your body. Take it before and every three months after initiating the 108 steps in this book. It will help track your progress.

Be sure to ask your health-care provider to check your blood work for inflammatory markers, including:

Tumor necrosis factor (TNF alpha)

Nuclear factor-kappa B (NF-kB)

Interleukins 22, 23, and 10

Prostaglandin E2

Leukotriene B4

Hs-CRP

MPO, or myeloperoxidase

Plac 2 (LpPLA2)

4. Ask Your Health Care Provider for a Body-Composition Test.

Your bathroom scale tells you how much you weigh. It does not reveal your ideal body weight. It does not measure the amount of fat versus muscle in your body. A healthy body has a healthy ratio of water, fat, bone, and muscle—what's known as a healthy body composition.

Because many of my patients don't realize that weight doesn't tell us about body composition, they often lament that while their clothes fit differently after starting a lifestyle change program and they have lost inches from their waistlines, they haven't lost much weight. It's likely that their body composition changed because they gained muscle, which weighs more than fat. And improved body composition should be the goal, not the number on the scale.

Here is a simple way to think about it: your body has both a fat component and a "fat-free" component. Your body fat also has two components: storage fat and essential fat. The fat in your bone marrow and nervous system is essential to good health. It is the fat your body needs to function normally. The rest is storage fat. That's the fat that fills your tissues in less than desirable ways. Your lean body mass is the weight of your muscles, bones, ligaments, tendons, and internal organs and includes the essential fat in these organs.

Body fat ranges for optimal health (18 to 30 percent for women and 15 to 20 percent for men) are based on those of the general population. Slightly lower body fat percentage is more desirable: 11 to 14 percent for men and 16 to 23 percent for women. Ranges may be lower in elite athletes, but keep in mind that normal body function may be affected if your body fat falls below the minimum level recommended for men (5 percent) and women (15 percent). For example, women athletes commonly stop menstruating when their body fat composition is below 15 percent.

Once you understand your body composition, you can set better goals for your ideal body weight, percent body fat, and lean body mass. And then you can develop a program to help achieve these goals using your body composition measurements to track your success.

The PROVE IT Study and the Role of Inflammation

A large study called PROVE IT evaluated the effect of high-dose statin therapy on individuals with heart disease.[1] Researchers were surprised to learn that those individuals who received the greatest benefit from statin therapy were those who also had the lowest levels of inflammation. In fact, even at the same LDL cholesterol level, those with less inflammation had fewer cardiovascular events!

The study strongly indicates that the potential benefit of statin therapy is less about lowering cholesterol and more about decreasing inflammation.

5. Identify Your Inflammation Triggers.

Your diet, sleep patterns, and other lifestyle behaviors can have a significant impact on inflammation. Brad, a much-loved veterinarian in his 50s, came to me because he was having atrial fibrillation, a condition in which the heart beats irregularly. Usually, we treat this condition with blood thinners, such as warfarin, and medications to regulate the heart rate. In some cases, we may do surgery or an ablation procedure. But Brad was not interested in these options. I asked him to start keeping a journal of when his heart beat irregularly and of what he was eating, drinking, or doing at the time.

We quickly learned that Brad had episodes of atrial fibrillation after eating sugar or foods high in simple carbohydrates. I explained that not only was sugar causing his irregular heartbeat, it was an important cause of inflammation. (We will discuss this in detail shortly.) Brad went on a low-glycemic diet and stopped drinking simple sugars such as fruit juice and soda; these are liquid sugar and a source of unneeded calories. He ate only complex carbohydrates like quinoa and brown rice and eliminated white foods such as cereal, white bread, and potatoes. In addition, we started Brad on magnesium, an important mineral and micronutrient known to prevent arrhythmia.

That was four years ago, and Brad has had no further episodes of atrial fibrillation since changing his diet and adding a magnesium supplement.

Carrying extra weight around the midline is a less recognized cause of inflammation. We call these fat cells VAT, or visceral adipose tissue, and they line our organs and fill our abdominal cavity. This fat cannot be removed by techniques such as liposuction. Abdominal fat is actually an endocrine organ, producing chemicals or cytokines that are released into the blood. These cytokines raise blood pressure, cause inflammation, and lead to diabetes, heart disease, and cancer. Inflammatory cytokines are even linked to depression!

Sleep is another factor in inflammation. When you don't get enough sleep or have irregular sleep patterns, the body triggers a defense system that leads to inflammation. Researchers at Emory University in Atlanta found that sleep deprivation or just poor sleep quality increases inflammation. Sleep apnea, a sleep disorder in which people snore and then stop breathing, often hundreds of times a night, is another hidden source of inflammation.

Take a Quick Inventory of Your Diet and Body

Are you consuming pro-inflammatory foods, such as sugar? Do you have symptoms of arthritis, indigestion, heartburn, gas, bloating, muscle aches, and brain fog? Do you walk 10,000 steps a day or get 30 minutes of exercise? Do you feel rested upon waking in the morning, or are you still tired? Is your sleep fragmented and disturbed?

Finally, how do you cope with stress and tension? Do you feel overwhelmed and in survival mode? Inflammation is linked to each and every one of these. Once you identify your triggers, you can start to make positive changes to put the fire out.

6. Know Whether You Have a Food Allergy or a Food Sensitivity.

Many people use the terms "food sensitivity" and "food allergy" interchangeably, but they are very different. The reactions are driven by distinct immune response factors in the body. Sensitivities are caused by immune system cells called IgG (immunoglobulin G), while allergies are caused by IgE (immunoglobulin E).

While nearly a third of people in the United States believe they have a food allergy, only 4 percent of teens and adults have a true food allergy. The eight most common food allergens are dairy, eggs, peanuts, tree nuts, soy, wheat and other gluten-containing grains, fish, and shellfish. Citrus fuits are another common allergen.

So how does this translate to everyday life?

- **A food allergy happens quickly and is an emergency.** An allergic reaction can occur anywhere from minutes to an hour after eating or even touching the offending food. The immune system sees the food as an attack on the body, and IgE antibodies spring into action. (Remember: *E* is for emergency.) The body releases histamine, causing symptoms ranging from mild itching and hives to severe anaphylaxis, an intense allergic reaction that involves the nose, throat, lungs, and gastrointestinal tract. Food allergy requires immediate medical assistance to stop the reaction; many people with true food allergies carry epinephrine pens for such emergencies.

- **Food sensitivity takes a slower, more gradual course.** The immune factor involved here is IgG (remember *G* for gradual). Among the most common symptoms of food sensitivity are fatigue, trouble sleeping, mental fogginess, mood changes, irritability, anger, headache, joint pain, skin irritation, and rashes. Nasal congestion, postnasal drip, sinus infections, and ear infections can also be related to food sensitivity, as can arthritis, muscle stiffness, and joint pain. Gas, bloating, and diarrhea are symptoms as well. Common culprits include dairy, gluten, corn, soy, tree nuts, eggs, shellfish, and citrus.

You'll know right away if you have a food allergy. However, you may not recognize when you have a food sensitivity, even though your body is engaged in an ongoing battle to clear an invading toxin from your system. Food sensitivity is one of the causes of low-grade chronic inflammation—and its long-term consequences can be enormous. This inflammation may affect any organ and cause symptoms including arthritis, skin irritation, intestinal discomfort, and even brain fog. If you have a chronic health issue that does not respond to treatment, you may have a food sensitivity.

Recently, a high-powered corporate executive named Bob came to my office for a consultation. Bob had been having chest pain, and his wife was concerned about his heart. I was not happy to hear that Bob was receiving monthly steroid injections from his primary care physician. He explained: "Dr. G., if I do not take those injections, my joints ache so badly that I can't get out of bed in the morning. I can't even walk. And then I get this horrible skin rash that everyone can see. I can't go into a board meeting covered in a skin rash, so every month, I have steroid injections."

Bob's symptoms, paired with his frequent sinus infections, immediately caused me to suspect gluten sensitivity. I ordered a few simple blood tests, and though Bob was adamant that he was not sensitive to gluten, the tests showed otherwise. Within months of becoming gluten-free, all of Bob's symptoms resolved.

A patient named Valerie also had frequent sinus infections. One year, she took six 10-day courses of antibiotics, but when that proved unsuccessful, her physician recommended sinus surgery. At her mom's advice, she came to see me for an appointment. I suggested to Valerie that she avoid the most common food allergens for a few weeks and placed her on a diet free of gluten, dairy, corn, and soy.

About six months later, Valerie came in for a follow-up appointment. She said, "I need your help, Dr. G. I am being dropped from my insurance company for being a noncompliant patient because I never had the recommended sinus surgery. I tried to explain about the elimination diet and how I was cured of my sinus problems, but they would not listen. By the way, it was dairy all along." Naturally, I wrote a letter for Valerie, and she was reinstated by her insurance company.

How can *you* know if you are sensitive to certain foods? You can ask your health-care provider for a food sensitivity blood test, but you can also start by trying a simple elimination diet.

The Connection between Migraines and Gluten Sensitivity: A Study

The first randomized control trial to assess diet restriction in migraine headaches was published in *Headache* in 2010. Compared with baseline, those individuals who had IgG food sensitivity testing followed by diet restriction had a statistically reduced number of headache days.

Other studies have demonstrated links between migraine headaches, wine, and cheese. In 2013, a study published in *Headache* reported a higher prevalence of migraine headaches among individuals with celiac disease and gluten sensitivity.

7. Find Your Food Sensitivities with the Elimination Diet.

The elimination diet is a tool I use routinely in my practice to ascertain if food sensitivity is the underlying cause of sinus congestion, headaches, joint and muscle pain, irritable bowel syndrome, mental fogginess, and a host of other symptoms.

I love milk. If I could, I would drink a quart a day. I stopped drinking milk when my joints began to ache. Since I was too young to have arthritis, I started an elimination diet to see if my symptoms improved. When I eliminated dairy, the inflammation in my joints disappeared.

The concept of the elimination diet is simple: remove suspect food categories from your diet and see if you feel better. You can eliminate one or more foods at a time. If you have multiple or severe symptoms, you should eliminate the most common food irritants—dairy, gluten, corn, soy, tree nuts, citrus, shellfish, and egg—for two full weeks, with no exceptions. Even a bite or two of a potential offender can skew your results.

Be sure to eliminate not only the food itself but also any other foods that may include that ingredient. Dairy, for example, includes all milk, cream, cheese, cottage cheese, yogurt, ice cream, frozen yogurt, and butter. It even includes milk chocolate. If a food contains butter or whey as an ingredient, it's also off-limits.

If you are eliminating gluten, remember that it is in wheat, spelt, rye, barley, malt, and cereals. Condiments such as ketchup, mayonnaise, and mustard all contain vinegar that frequently comes from wheat or corn and so will contain trace amounts of gluten. You have to read the labels carefully. You will be surprised how many foods contain wheat, soy, or corn. If you are sensitive to oats, avoid them unless the package specifies they are gluten-free.

Getting Started

First, make a list of foods that do and do not contain the ingredients you want to eliminate. A nutritionist or reliable online resource can help. Then stock your house with the foods that are allowed.

It's a good idea to eat at home during this time so you can more easily control the ingredients in your diet. If you are eliminating protein sources such as soy, nuts, and eggs, talk with your health-care provider about adding a high-nutrient protein supplement such as a rice- or pea-protein meal replacement. Peas and rice are hypoallergenic and usually well tolerated.

Drink plenty of filtered water, and don't exercise too strenuously. Your body is clearing toxins, and it needs to heal. Instead of doing lengthy workouts or heavy strength training, take a walk outside for about 10 minutes or do gentle yoga.

Keep a journal during the process and note how you feel as you begin to eliminate and then reintroduce foods. It can be hard to remember how you felt a few days ago when you have your usual day-to-day activities to handle. Writing everything down will give you time to focus and help you pay close attention to withdrawal symptoms, cravings, improvements in your health problems, and your general well-being. If you completed the medical symptom questionnaire earlier, do it again and compare the results.

What to Expect: The First Two Weeks

Day 1: Eliminate all or some of the common food irritants.

Days 2 to 7: Your symptoms may seem to get worse and flare up. This is to be expected as you clear your body of toxins. If you have aches and pains or find yourself craving the foods you have eliminated, stick it out and be strong. These are all normal withdrawal symptoms as your body cleanses itself. (In Traditional Chinese Medicine, this is called a healing crisis.)

Days 8 to 14: Your symptoms should improve. If they do, then you know that at least one of the tested food groups is causing your symptoms.

The Big Question: Which Food Is It?

The only way to know *which* of the food categories is causing your problem is to start adding them back in, one at a time.

Day 15: Try eating a small amount of one food category at breakfast, lunch, and dinner. Then stop eating it again. How does your body react?

Day 16 to 18: Continue paying attention to the signals your body is sending. Do your joints hurt again? Is your mental fogginess back? Are your sinuses congested?

Repeat these steps with each of the food categories you've eliminated. After you reintroduce a food and see how your body reacts, it's important that you don't add it back again until you have tested all food categories. It is common to be sensitive to several foods, and this will help you determine which ones are problematic.

Elimination Diet Shortcuts

Giving up the foods you love can be challenging until you realize how much better you feel. Remember the most common food sensitivities: dairy, gluten, corn, soy, tree nuts, citrus, and egg. However, if eliminating all food categories for two weeks seems overwhelming, start with dairy and gluten. These are the two most common causes of food sensitivity and are most linked to arthritis, brain fog, stomach/intestinal discomfort, and sinus congestion.

You can also ask yourself which foods you can't live without—these are frequently the foods to which you are sensitive and the ones you eat the most. If you are still having symptoms, then eliminate the other food groups one at a time. After you are off of a food for six months, you may decide to reintroduce it slowly and monitor how you feel.

If arthritis is one of your main symptoms, eliminate foods from the nightshade family as well: tomato, cayenne, peppers, paprika, tomatillo, eggplant, and potatoes.

For a step-by-step guide to the elimination diet, including common substitutions, tips, a shopping list, and menu ideas, please see Appendix B.

8. *Control Your Blood Pressure Naturally.*

I can't stress this enough: The best way to control your blood pressure is to decrease your weight, eat a healthy diet, perform regular exercise and adequate sleep, and transform your response to stress and tension. Studies confirm that this body-mind-spirit approach works.

- **Lose weight.** Eleven clinical trials have shown that for every one kilogram of weight lost, systolic blood pressure drops by 1.6 mmHg and diastolic blood pressure drops by 1.6 mmHg. If you lose 10 kilograms (22 pounds), you would decrease systolic blood pressure by 16 points! Weight loss is the only treatment that can produce these results.

- **Exercise regularly.** It is one of the best ways to lose weight, and it also lowers your triglycerides, blood sugar, and LDL cholesterol. A combination of daily aerobic exercise with strength training can decrease blood pressure by 10 to 15 mmHg systolic and 5 to 10 mmHg diastolic.

  The Council of Clinical Cardiology recommends 40 minutes to 1 hour of aerobic exercise (such as brisk walking, swimming, jogging, cycling, or any activity that raises the heart rate and keeps it elevated) every day, and strength training at least three times per week.

- **Get proper sleep.** You should wake up feeling refreshed in the morning. If you snore, wake up multiple times during the night and/or feel sleepy during the day, you may have sleep apnea. Make sure your health-care provider checks you for this common cause of high blood pressure.

For specific recommendations for dietary changes and supplements to decrease high blood pressure, please see Chapters 4 and 5.

• ● •

CHAPTER 2

Your Genes Do Not Determine Your Destiny— You Do

On June 26, 2000, President Bill Clinton stood with scientists J. Craig Venter and Francis Collins to announce the completion of the Human Genome Project. For the first time, all the genes in the human body—the entire genome—were sequenced and mapped. What a remarkable day in our history!

While the genome actually had far fewer genes than researchers had anticipated, the number of variations of the genes was far greater than anyone expected: more than three million. In a nutshell, human beings are 99 percent genetically identical. It's the other 1 percent that determines our individuality. These variations define how we look and how we metabolize medications, toxins, and other substances. Our 1 percent is what makes each of us unique!

Researchers have continued to discover the many ways in which these variations make us unique and, most important, how they are relevant to disease.

9. Meet Your Microbiome.

It may be unsettling to learn that you have hundreds of different types of tiny microbes living all over your body. Think of these cells as flora—living organisms that reside in your mouth, nose, skin, stomach, intestinal tract, and just about everywhere else. The human microbiome consists of the genes or genetic material that these cells harbor.

These different types and species of microbes interact and communicate with each other. Many are quite promiscuous as well, exchanging genetic material with each other and even with some of our own cells. The good news is that our microbiomes help keep us healthy.

Each of us is a complete "walking ecosystem" just as biologically complex as any rainforest ecosystem. Scientists are just beginning to learn about this complexity due to recent developments in technology that allow them to study the genetic signatures of microbes directly. Prior to this, microbiologists could study only the microbes they could grow on petri dishes. Now they are in a huge rush to catch up on microbiology research using the new genetic sequencing technology.

A few discoveries have already been made. For one, only a very small percentage of bacteria species and strains cause disease. Most bacteria that live in and on us are either completely harmless or beneficial. Some bacteria produce essential vitamins for us, such as biotin, vitamin B12, and vitamin K2.

It is also thought that a diverse and healthy microbial ecosystem in our bodies essentially "crowds out" harmful bacteria, taking up the nutrients that the bad bacteria would use to grow and produce harmful toxins. In a sense, the enormous, complex microbial community living inside us generally looks out for our health and tries to keep us healthy—after all, if we die, they die!

In addition, many studies have started to show that the microbial ecosystem's composition and diversity are associated with obesity, inflammation levels, diabetes, and even mood disorders and autism. For example, obesity has been found to be associated with intestinal microbiota. The microbiota of obese individuals is more efficient at harvesting energy (i.e., calories), which can slow down metabolism. Other studies have shown that transplanting healthy microbial samples from one person to another can result in improvement of insulin sensitivity, which is the body's ability to transport sugar from the bloodstream into muscle.

Fecal transplant, the transfer of feces from one individual to another, has become standard medical practice for certain disorders, such as the deadly infection *Clostridium (C.) difficile*. Fortunately, a fecal transplant isn't required to reap these benefits. Research has shown that the microbiota of the gut also can be influenced by dietary interventions.

We've known for a long time that eating a plant-based diet high in fiber and nutrients contributes to our health. Scientists have recently discovered that legumes and vegetables actually feed the good bacteria in our bodies, which produce antioxidants and chemical signals that reduce harmful inflammation. Therefore, it is important to treat your microbes to dark leafy greens, beans, lentils, and other high-fiber plant foods such as broccoli, cabbage, kale, and all the cruciferous vegetables.

The Good News on Good Bacteria

It's an exciting time for researchers in this field, and we can look forward to astounding breakthroughs and, potentially, new kinds of natural, microbial-based treatments for many diseases. A perfect example is probiotic therapy. Probiotics are bacteria known to change the gut environment. Research has shown that probiotics can ease symptoms of irritable bowel syndrome and colitis, as well as help to prevent antibiotic-induced diarrhea. This is why your doctor may advise that you eat yogurt or take a probiotic supplement while you are taking an antibiotic.

Laboratory testing can also be conducted to assess your microbiome and determine the best probiotics for you. In addition, these tests can look for gut inflammation markers (calprotectin and secretory IgA) as well as pathogens and parasites.

10. Understand Your Unique Genetic Variability— and Apply It To Life.

Hollywood movies have completely misrepresented the words "mutant" and "mutation," leading many to think that a mutation invariably produces some kind of green, slimy monster.

In reality, a mutation is an alteration in a genetic code. Sometimes mutations produce adverse effects, but more often they produce no observable effects, and in some cases, a mutation may actually be beneficial.

Think of a genetic code as being a string of As, Cs, Ts, and Gs. Each letter represents a nucleotide: A for adenine, C for cytosine, T for thymine, and G for guanine. Their combinations form words, sentences, and paragraphs that code for the formation of specific proteins. So, you can think of a mutation as a typo or a misspelling in the genetic code. Here's what I mean. If you changed the spelling of the word "center" to "centre," for example, the meaning would be the same. But if you changed the word "cat" to "cot," Dr. Seuss would have written a much different book called *The Cot in the Hat.*

The same thing happens in genetics. A single letter change can mean nothing, or it can alter the function of the protein that a gene codes for. The technical term for this is "single nucleotide polymorphism" (SNP), or "single nucleotide variation" (SNV). The latter case is where it might affect health.

A common genetic polymorphism is Factor V Leiden. Individuals with Factor V Leiden are more likely to have blood clots, which can form in any part of the body. Most commonly, people develop clots in their legs; the clots can then break off and travel to other parts of the body, such as the lungs. In addition, women with Factor V Leiden have two to three times the number of miscarriages in comparison to women who do not have this mutation.

Understanding this genetic variant is very important, since women who carry this mutation may be more prone to blood clots when prescribed birth control and hormone replacement therapy. The chance of developing a blood clot depends on the genes you inherit from your parents.

By understanding how genetic variations can affect your health, you can make smarter lifestyle choices. You can start by speaking with your health-care provider about genetic testing. Ask if you should be tested for BRCA1 and BRCA2 if you have a family history of breast or ovarian cancer. Ask about Factor V Leiden if you have a history of blood clots or miscarriage. There are many other genetic variants that require only a simple blood test or saliva sample to identify.

I routinely use epigenetic testing to understand how my patients respond to stress, how they metabolize vitamin D, and how they process folate and vitamin B12. When it comes to the lining of the blood vessel, called the endothelium, genes that lead to the formation of nitric oxide are critically important—and this can be assessed through genetic testing.

The "Breast Cancer" Gene

You have probably heard about the BRCA1 and BRCA2 genes. These two BRCA proteins are among more than 100 different kinds that help ensure correct DNA replication during cell division. Think of BRCAs as part of a class of proteins that serve as DNA proofreaders, spell checkers, and autocorrect tools. When these proofreading proteins encounter DNA damage, they either repair it (correct the spelling) or, if the damage is too extensive to correct, tell the cell its code can't be repaired and so it needs to undergo a preprogrammed suicide (sacrifice itself for the greater benefit of the entire body).

There are people who have mutations in either the BRCA1 or BRCA2 genes that cause their cells to produce proofreading proteins that do not function properly. As a result, their cells may go on to freely replicate damaged DNA without the benefit of proofreading and correction. Without proofreading and correction, the DNA code gets more and more corrupted with every cell division. There is a higher risk that eventually, a mutation may arise in a gene that codes for a protein that tells cells to grow and divide. If that happens, then those cells may start growing rapidly out of control. Even worse, those cells can accumulate even more DNA mutations at an accelerated pace. The result is complete chaos in DNA code spelling and cell reproduction. This is often how cancers start and progress.

However, contrary to what you see in the media, there is no such thing as a "breast cancer" gene. Everyone, both men and women, has two copies each of the BRCA1 and BRCA2 genes. Some people who have mutations in either one or both of those genes that can produce defective proofreading proteins are more highly susceptible to developing certain cancers—particularly breast cancer.

11. Understand How Your Environment Influences Your DNA.

We are born with a certain set of genes—our DNA. It's our individual book of life, what makes us unique. Changes in our environment—and how we live our life—can cause changes in our genes. This is why identical twins may grow up with very different characteristics and life outcomes.

Let's take a quick trip back to 10th-grade biology class to understand how this happens. At conception, we inherit 23 chromosomes from each parent. The chromosomes are made up of DNA, which is tightly coiled around proteins. DNA carries information to our cells.

We have two copies of each gene in every cell; we inherit one copy from each parent. Each cell expresses only a portion of its genes, and the remainder of the gene is turned off or repressed. This is a normal process. (Imagine what would happen, for example, if genes that produce muscle tissue were expressed in the brain.) When we turn a gene on or off, our bodies produce different kinds of proteins.

How we look and act results from the interaction of our genes and our environment. This interaction occurs through the *epigenome*. The epigenome includes all the elements that are capable of turning genes on and off. This discovery is one of the most exciting breakthroughs in genetic research. We now know that chemical changes in our environment can regulate gene activity and change gene expression. The prefix *epi* means "above" in Greek; epigenetic changes are on or attached to the DNA. Our genes can react to environmental changes very quickly. As such, environmental influences such as pollution, tobacco use, or diet can affect which proteins our genes produce.

There is no question that major medical conditions from Alzheimer's disease to type 2 diabetes to heart disease and even some cancers are influenced by environmental factors. Our chances of developing them can be increased or decreased by how we live our lives.

What happens to your genes when you eat a vegan diet and live a healthy, active lifestyle? According to a prostate cancer study led by Dr. Dean Ornish, men who made these and other healthy lifestyle choices were able to down-regulate more than 500 cancer genes. Think about that. How we live, what we eat, how we manage stress, our exposure level to toxins—these things and a host of other environmental factors all influence our epigenetics. They define which genes we turn on or off and how the story in our book of life develops.

12. Know Your Mutagens!

Mutagens are anything that brings about a change in a cell's genetic code, or DNA. They are all around us and come in many forms, from X-ray radiation to tobacco smoke. Many mutagens are also carcinogens. How can we limit our exposure to these DNA-altering substances? First, you need to identify them:

— **Combustion products.** These are powerful sources of mutagens—tobacco smoke in particular. Anything that produces carbon soot is likely to also produce a class of compounds called polycyclic aromatic hydrocarbons (PAHs). The high prevalence of cancer among chimney sweepers demonstrates the link between soot, PAHs, and cancers.

— **Chemical mutagens.** There are many strong chemical mutagens, but one we are frequently exposed to is acetaldehyde. For example, when your body eliminates alcohol from your system, it converts it into acetaldehyde. Grain alcohol, or ethanol, is not nearly as damaging to your DNA as the acetaldehyde it's converted to.

— **Ionizing radiation.** Another common source of mutagens is ionizing radiation. *Ionizing* means that the radiation is energetic enough to remove electrons from atoms and molecules. Much of the ultraviolet light in sunlight and tanning booths is ionizing, as is radiation from medical procedures such as X-rays and CT scans.

Most medical professionals now have highly sophisticated equipment intended to keep radiation exposure as low as possible and far below dangerous limits. If you have a life-threatening emergency and require an immediate X-ray or CT scan, don't hesitate to get one. Still, it is never a good idea to get radiation exposure that's not medically necessary.

The FDA has launched an initiative to reduce unnecessary radiation exposure, beginning with CT and nuclear scans. In addition to monitoring equipment safety and establishing criteria for radiation use, the FDA is encouraging consumers to keep track of their personal medical imaging history.

— **Radon gas.** This is another potent source of radiation exposure. Radon is a breakdown product of uranium, a natural radioactive material found in bricks, rocks, soil, and concrete. It is regarded as the second leading cause of lung cancer behind cigarette smoke. Radon gas is odorless and colorless, and it typically seeps into our homes (especially basements and first floors) from cracks in building foundations.

— **Free radicals.** For most of us, however, the greatest exposure to mutagens is simply normal respiration in our body's cells. Although oxygen is an essential requirement for life, it can become damaging to the human body when it becomes a free radical.

Free radicals are single atoms or groups of atoms that have one or more unpaired electrons. (Free radicals derived from oxygen are known as reactive oxygen species.) They can be derived either from normal metabolic processes in the human body or from external sources such as exposure to ozone, X-rays, air pollution, cigarette smoking, and industrial chemicals.

Free radicals are highly reactive and damage biologically important molecules such as DNA, lipids, proteins, and carbohydrates, causing cell damage. In fact, atherosclerosis (also known as "hardening" of the arteries) results from free-radical reactions between lipids (fats) from food, the arterial wall, and blood serum, which create substances that induce endothelial cell injury and lead to plaque formation.

Because we breathe oxygen and our bodies need it to produce energy, our cells produce an endless supply of errant free radicals. *Oxidative stress* is the term used to describe the imbalance between free-radical formation and our body's antioxidant defenses. An antioxidant is a stable molecule that can donate an electron to a free radical and neutralize it, thereby reducing its capacity to damage DNA and other cells. Antioxidants are affectionately known as free-radical scavengers.

13. Minimize the Negative Effects of Mutagens.

Exposure to mutagens is inevitable. But you can take these steps to minimize your exposure and ameliorate their effects:

- **Combustion products.** As a rule of thumb, avoid smoke of any kind, as well as charred foods. Of course, avoid tobacco smoke, which not only contains PAHs but also high concentrations of hundreds of known mutagens and carcinogens.

- **Chemical mutagens.** Limit alcohol use. Excessive alcohol use is associated with higher risks of many cancers, including liver, breast, esophageal, pancreatic, and colon cancers.

- **Ionizing radiation.** Review the topic of radiation-emitting products on the FDA website at www.fda. org, and then make note of all radiation procedures you have. Discuss excessive or unnecessary medical radiation exposure concerns during routine visits with your health-care provider. Ask if a nonradiation procedure can be used for testing instead. Stay out of tanning beds, and avoid excessive exposure to strong sunlight.

- **Radon gas.** Check the radon gas measurements in your home. You can have the test performed by a professional or use a kit found in many home improvement stores. Radon levels in your home can vary from day to day and season to season, so it is wise to measure levels for at least three months.

- **Free radicals.** The best aids in your body's defenses against free radicals are the antioxidants found in fruits, vegetables, and many spices. Make the right food choices; strong antioxidant activities have been found in berries, cherries, citrus, prunes, olives, and tea. Take potent antioxidant supplements such as vitamin C, vitamin E, and melatonin. Also ask your health-care provider about taking a blood test to check your antioxidant levels.

14. Take the Right Amount of Medicine for Your Genome.

Whenever we take a medication, vitamin, or supplement, our bodies consider it a foreign substance, almost like an intruder. Enzymes found primarily in our liver and intestines recognize these foreign substances and methodically convert them to a water-soluble form that can be excreted from the body via our kidneys or liver until they are eliminated.

This is why we typically follow a dosing schedule for medication (e.g., twice a day for five days). By prescribing specific amounts of medication at regular intervals, physicians aim to keep the level of a drug in our blood within a therapeutic range even while our body tries to eliminate the drug from our system. It's a continual tug-of-war.

It's common sense that a 95-pound woman may need a smaller dose of medication than a 350-pound man to produce the same safe, desired effect. Body mass or weight alone is, however, a very rough, crude estimate for medication and supplement dosing. We now know that our genes play a significant role in our response to medication, vitamins, and supplements: enter pharmacogenomics. This emerging field studies ways to personalize drug selection and dosing specific to a person's unique genetic makeup for maximum effectiveness with minimum side effects, and it may change the way we take medications and supplements forever.

Historically, drug manufacturers and their pharmacologists have developed dosing guidelines around an individual's body size and mass (height, weight, and body surface area). However, all the enzymes responsible for metabolizing and eliminating drugs from our bodies are encoded by our genes, which can vary greatly from person to person. This is why a particular dose might be too low to be effective for one person, yet so high as to cause toxic side effects in another.

If you take prescription medications or simply want to understand how your body metabolizes medication, ask your healthcare provider to consider testing your pharmacogenetics. Many companies offer pharmacogenetic testing. Not only can it help to pinpoint your metabolism of medication, which aids in dose selection, but it may also help prevent unnecessary side effects. In individuals with cardiovascular disease, testing can be done to assess the metabolism of medications such as clopidogrel (Plavix), a common platelet inhibitor; statin therapy; and response to beta blockers—just to name a few.

A Better Way to Establish Dosing

Many companies can now assess your response to medication based on your genes. In this important and emerging area, it is becoming possible to determine what medication and supplements are best for an individual challenged with depression or anxiety.

Another example of the potential of this technology is with warfarin, a potent blood thinner given to people with artificial heart valves and an irregular heart rhythm called atrial fibrillation. Physicians have historically guessed the starting dose of warfarin for their patients. As a result, it has been difficult to get the level correct quickly. Now we can use genetic testing to help us determine whether an individual needs a high or low starting dose. This not only helps us to determine the proper level quickly but also helps to prevent side effects such as bleeding and clot formation.

• ● •

CHAPTER 3

You Are What You Eat

In the early days of my career, in the 1990s, it did not faze me to see a patient in the ICU eating a roast beef and mayo sandwich on white bread. In fact, this was a common sight. Like most physicians back then, I didn't understand the relationship between nutrition and heart disease prevention.

Today, numerous studies confirm the role of diet in disease prevention. We know now that certain foods harm while other foods heal. Hot dogs harm. Hemp seeds heal. Refined grains harm. Whole grains heal.

In 2010, studies found that women who ate meat—particularly red and cured meat—prior to being diagnosed with ovarian cancer were less likely to have a positive outcome. Another study found that approximately 100,000 cancer deaths a year were related to being overweight. Obesity has been linked to the consumption of excess calories and refined or simple carbohydrates, exposure to toxins in the environment, a lack of physical activity, and a high stress load.

In 2015, the World Health Organization reported that hot dogs, sausage, and other processed meats have been classified in the same cancer-causing category as tobacco smoking and asbestos.

So how can you use this information to optimize your own health?

15. Think of Food as Information for Your Body.

Everything we eat and drink is metabolized, broken down, and carried into our cells through our bloodstream. When we have lunch, our cells don't see a spinach salad. They see folate, beta-carotene, and iron. If we add eggs or almonds to the salad, they also see protein in the form of good fat.

These nutrients in the food we eat send instructions to our cells. Some foods instruct our genes to produce proteins that prevent heart disease, Alzheimer's disease, arthritis, and inflammation. Other foods—such as those high in refined flour and sugar—signal our genes to produce proteins that result in arthritis, back pain, shoulder pain, heart disease, and memory loss.

There is much wisdom in the Ayurvedic proverb that states, "With the right food, medicine is of no need. With the wrong food, medicine is of no use." Today's research validates what generations before us knew: food is medicine.

The China Study

The China Study, still considered one of the most comprehensive nutrition books ever published, analyzed 50 diseases in rural China and compared the food in China with the food in the United States. Here's what we learned:

- Fat intake was twice as high in the United States as in China.

- Fiber intake from fruits and vegetables was three times lower in the United States.

- The consumption of animal protein—such as beef, pork and lamb—was 90 percent higher in the United States.

- Heart disease death rates were 16 times greater in the United States for men and five times greater for women.

- Cancer, osteoporosis, diabetes, and high blood pressure were more prevalent in the United States.

16. Avoid Foods that Lead to Inflammation.

If you've done the elimination diet that I discuss in Chapter 1 and Appendix B, you now have an idea of your food sensitivities. Know that, along with foods that you personally are sensitive to, there are certain food categories that can lead to inflammation in your body. In general, it's best to avoid the following:

— **Added sugar.** This includes white sugar, brown sugar, raw sugar, corn syrup, molasses, agave, dextrose, fructose, maltose, and sucrose. If you have any health problems linked to inflammation—such as heart disease, memory loss, or arthritis—eliminate sugar first. You should not have more than 20 grams of added sugar a day. (Some foods, such as fruit, contain naturally occuring sugar. This is not an added sugar, and it is OK to eat two or three servings of fruit a day.)

— **Certain cooking oils.** Steer clear of oils that are high in omega-6 fatty acids and those sensitive to heat, creating potentially tissue-damaging oxidation. Avoid cottonseed, sesame, corn, safflower, and sunflower oil. These heavily processed oils are usually found in fast foods and processed foods.

— **Trans fats.** Most fats in this category are artificially created, and they increase bad cholesterol (LDL) and lower good cholesterol (HDL). Not surprisingly, these damaging fats are found in deep-fried foods, fast foods, and commercially prepared baked goods. Always avoid products that list "partially hydrogenated oil" as an ingredient.

— **Milk.** Lactose intolerance—the inability of the digestive system to tolerate milk—affects 60 percent of the world's population. While typical symptoms include upset stomach, diarrhea, gas, and bloating, milk is also a common cause of inflammation-related arthritis and skin rashes. You can try substituting unsweetened coconut or almond milk.

— **Cured meats and red meats.** These can trigger inflammation through a substance called neu5Gc, which is a sugar molecule found in meats—mainly beef, pork, and lamb. The body sees neu5Gc as a foreign invader and attacks it with antibodies, which is an inflammatory response; chronic inflammation is known to promote tumor growth. Research at the University of California at San Diego demonstrated spontaneous cancer development in mice fed neu5Gc. I suggest avoiding cured and red meat.

— **Heavy drinking.** Overconsumption of alcohol is linked to inflammation of the esophagus and can lead to esophageal and laryngeal cancers. Heavy drinking affects the liver as well, leading to cirrhosis and alcohol-induced hepatitis. Alcohol is also fairly high in empty calories and can only be broken down slowly by the liver. Drinking alcohol leads to the conversion of carbohydrates to fat. These fat cells deregulate sugar metabolism and cause insulin resistance.

Portion Control: Limiting alcohol consumption to one four-ounce glass of wine per day is generally recommended for men and fewer than three to four glasses a week for women. For many, alcohol is a coping strategy to deal with stress, so before you pour yourself a glass of wine, consider other ways to unwind, such as a walk around the neighborhood, meditation, or calling a friend.

— **Refined grains.** Research shows that refined grains lead to inflammation. Avoid white grains, and don't be fooled by color. Some dark brown breads are actually refined. Don't choose breads labeled "wheat" or "multigrain." Only buy 100 percent whole-grain products.

— **Artificial food additives.** Additives such as monosodium glutamate (MSG) and aspartame activate inflammation. These additives are found only in packaged or processed foods. Artificial additives or sweeteners are never recommended, even in small amounts.

17. Uncover Hidden Sources of Salt in Your Diet.

When I first met Tom, 37, I was surprised that he was taking three medications for high blood pressure. Tom was tall and thin, outwardly happy, and actively playing basketball for fun. Despite laboratory tests that showed he was in overall good health, he still had high blood pressure.

I asked Tom to tell me about his life. "I want to know what you eat, whom you eat with, what you drink, how you prepare your food. I want to review your entire day," I insisted.

I didn't have to dig very deep to get to the underlying cause of his high blood pressure. Tom was drinking 15 bottles of electrolyte drinks a day; these drinks are filled with sodium! Tom's presciption was simple: give up the electrolyte drinks. Once he did so, his blood pressure returned to normal.

The sodium found in salt is vital to our health. It maintains the balance of fluids in our bodies and keeps our muscles working properly. Yet most Americans consume way more than they need. Our bodies require only about 500 milligrams of sodium a day to function; the average American takes in 6 to 10 times that amount.

In 30 percent of people, a high-sodium diet is associated with high blood pressure. The goal is to keep your sodium ingestion to 1500 milligrams or less per day, so it's critical that you carefully consider the packaged and canned food you eat.

One little cup of canned chicken noodle soup has 1,400 milligrams of sodium. That's nearly all the sodium you should have for the entire day. If you eat the whole can, you have had about 2,800 milligrams. Two slices of white bread have 340 milligrams of sodium. Three ounces of ham have 1,000 milligrams of sodium. Just about every item on a restaurant menu contains salt. All too often, a shocking amount.

What's the answer? Eat whole foods. One cup of unsalted almonds has 1 milligram of sodium. A whole mango has 5 milligrams. So pay attention to how much sodium you are eating. Remember, it should be no more than 1,500 milligrams a day. An easy way to keep track is with one of the many available apps that help you add up your sodium throughout the day.

You can also try a salt substitute, such as NoSalt, which can actually lower your blood pressure (but if your blood potassium level is high, it is better to avoid NoSalt since it contains potassium chloride instead of sodium chloride).

However, it is not as simple as sodium being the bad guy. It's important to note that foods high in sodium are often low in potassium, an important mineral in lowering blood pressure. Usually, when we eat a high-sodium diet we are also eating less potassium-containing foods. It is the sodium-to-potassium ratio that is truly important.

Green leafy vegetables are high in potassium. But many foods and drinks contain surprisingly high amounts of sodium, so you may be consuming much more than you realize. If you eat whole, unpackaged foods, you are most likely eating a healthy high-potassium, low-sodium diet.

In addition, avoid black licorice and black jelly beans. Although they do not contain sodium, they contain a substance that causes salt retention, which can result in high blood pressure.

A Look at the DASH II Diet

The National Heart, Lung, and Blood Institute did an amazing study of a diet called the DASH II. They studied three groups of people. The control group ate a typical American diet with more than 3,000 milligrams of sodium a day. The intermediate group restricted sodium intake to 2,300 milligrams. The third group cut the sodium down to 1,500 milligrams per day. Remember, our bodies need just 500 milligrams, so even the low-sodium group was eating three times the required sodium.

Even so, this third group who ate just 1,500 milligrams of sodium per day reduced their systolic blood pressure by 11.5 mmHg and diastolic by 6.8 mmHg. That can make the difference between needing to take blood pressure medication or not.

Based on this research and many years of clinical practice, I recommend keeping daily sodium intake to less than 1,500 milligrams for individuals with high blood pressure.

18. Beware of "Fortified": The "Red Flag" in Food Labeling.

Next time you're at the grocery store, take a walk down the breakfast cereal aisle and scan the boxes. You'll see this phrase over and over again: "fortified with vitamins and minerals." Sounds healthy, right? Yet the word *fortified* is one of my red flags. If we have to fortify a food, it is usually because something was taken out, usually something good for you. These foods can also be referred to as *refined*.

Refining foods removes important vitamins and minerals. Refined white rice, for example, has been stripped of its nutrient value. White rice is milled rice that has had its husk, bran, and germ removed, so most of its fiber and nutrients are lost. This changes the way the rice looks, feels, and tastes. It also helps prevent it from spoiling, so you can keep it on the shelf longer with all the other processed and refined foods.

Food refinement strips out 85 percent of magnesium. This essential mineral prevents irregular heartbeats (known in cardiology as arrhythmia), helps us sleep, and keeps our bowels moving. Food refinement removes 77 percent of its thiamine, so if you don't get enough thiamine from food, you have to take a supplement. It's the same with iron—76 percent is removed in the refining process. But you need iron to make red blood cells. When we refine food, we also remove copper, zinc, calcium and just about every nutrient needed to build strong, healthy bones.

Whole, unrefined foods contain soluble fiber, which is a miracle food in my opinion. It binds the fatty acids in the intestine and pulls them out of the body. This helps to lower cholesterol and blood sugar. It also promotes regular bowel movements, which is especially helpful for people with diverticular disease and constipation. Finally, fiber blocks the quick absorption of sugar, which keeps blood sugar levels low.

Soluble fiber is found in all kinds of whole foods. Nutritious, functional foods don't need to be fortified. Substitute at least one processed or refined food in your diet with a whole food. Swap your fortified breakfast cereal for steel-cut oats, or eat quinoa instead of white. Always choose a whole fruit instead of fruit juice.

19. Avoid Pesticides—Buy Organic.

Is it really necessary to buy organic foods? This is one of the most common questions patients ask in my practice. It's also one of the easiest for me to answer.

First, you need to understand that the term *organic* describes the way agricultural products are grown and processed. The goal of organic farming is to avoid the use of chemicals such as synthetic fertilizers and pesticides, reduce pollution, and make the best use of resources such as soil and water.

Organic farmers don't use chemical pesticides to reduce pests; they use mulch and other natural products.

Organic farmers don't use chemical fertilizers. They rotate their crops to allow the soil to recover and regenerate. This supports the crops' growth without depleting the soil.

Organic farmers don't feed antibiotics or hormones to chicks and cows or keep them caged in crowded and unpleasant conditions. They feed their livestock organic feed and provide access to the outdoors.

So is it really necessary to choose organic foods, or just smart? Is organic worth the cost?

It's true that organic foods are generally more expensive, but for good reason. If you buy organic, you are getting natural fertilizers, not chemical. You are avoiding harmful hormones and antibiotics as well as foods that are genetically modified.

Because organic farmers also rotate their crops, their soil is less depleted of vital nutrients. Why is that? Well, if you grow corn in the same spot year after year, for example, it can deplete the soil of nitrogen and phosphorus, and rotating crops prevents this problem.

So, yes, for all these reasons, I tell my patients to buy organic foods and support organic farming whenever possible.

What if you can't afford organic?

Every year, the Environmental Working Group publishes its Dirty Dozen list of the top 12 fruits and vegetables that are most contaminated by pesticides. If you can't afford to buy all organic foods, you should aim for organic versions of these. Generally, if a food has thin skin, like strawberries, apples, peaches, spinach, and lettuce, you should buy it organic. If it has a thicker skin and you can peel it, like an onion, an avocado, a mango, or a pineapple, it may not be as important to buy it organic—but it's still better to do so.

Check out the Environmental Working Group's website at www.EWG.org. Download the latest Dirty Dozen and Clean Fifteen lists, and reference these lists when you shop.

How Do You Know If a Food Is Truly Organic?

Read the labels. The U.S. Department of Agriculture (USDA) National Organic Program requires all organic foods to meet strict government standards that regulate how foods must be grown and processed to be certified and labeled as organic. Producers who sell less than $5,000 a year in organic foods are exempt from the certification process but must still follow the USDA requirements.

A "100 percent organic" label indicates that all ingredients must be certified organic. "Organic" means that all agricultural ingredients in the product must be certified organic, but nonorganic ingredients may be used as well.

Be the way, *organic* is not the same as *natural*. There is no regulation for labeling something as natural. Only foods that are grown and processed according to USDA organic standards can be labeled organic. Look for the number 9 on your fruit and vegetable labels. An easy way to remember this is to think of the phrase, "9 is divine"!

20. Say No to GMO

How do you know if the foods you eat are genetically modified? It's not easy if you live in the United States. Only two states have passed laws requiring food labeling for Genetically Modified Organism (GMO) foods, which have had specific changes introduced into their DNA to produce a desired result, such as a deeper color, larger size, or greater resistance to pests.

GMO or genetically engineered (GE) food can be found in more than 75 percent of our food supply, says the Environmental Working Group (EWG). These foods, including corn, soy, and canola oils, are found in 70 percent of popular processed foods such as frozen meals and cereals. How safe are these foods? We just don't know. Their long-term safety has not been proven.

What's more, genetically modified crops are incredibly resistant to pesticides. The extensive use of pesticides generates super-pesticide-resistant weeds. The result is the need for more pesticides, leading to further food contamination. Pesticides are also deadly to butterflies and good insects.

While the pesticide-producing companies argue that genetic modification is needed to produce enough food to feed the world, this is far from true. GMO crops actually contribute to world hunger by undermining sustainability.

Major GMO-food-producing corporations are spending millions of dollars each year to lobby against food-labeling legislation. We don't have the luxury of waiting for government-mandated food labeling. We do have the ability to control what we eat.

There are some simple things that you can do right now to avoid GMOs:

- **Buy foods that are certified organic.** Organic foods not only are free of synthetic pesticides, but they are also free of GMO ingredients.

- **Look for the Non-GMO Project verified label.** Go to www.nongmoproject.org for more information.

- **Download the Shopper's Guide to Avoiding GE Food** at www.EWG.org.

- **Avoid sugar.** The majority of sugar in the United States comes from sugar beets, which are GMO. Pure cane sugar is non-GMO. (However, it's best to limit added sugars overall.)

- **Avoid corn grown in the United States (unless organic)** and read all ingredients. Corn appears as corn flour and corn meal, high-fructose corn syrup, cornstarch and corn oil, and masa.

- **Avoid soy (unless organic),** including products that contain soy proteins. Edamame, soybean oil, soy milk, soy flour, soy sauce, tofu, and soy lecithin have been made with GMO ingredients.

- **Avoid "vegetable" oil, canola oil, cottonseed oil, and corn oil.** To be safe, assume that most are GMO.

• ● •

CHAPTER 4

Nutrition for Good Health and Healing

The formula for good health starts with the foods you choose. Focus on eating healthful, functional foods and eliminating or minimizing inflammatory ones. Functional foods are those that have a specific purpose in the body. Fiber, for example, lowers blood sugar and cholesterol. Dark green vegetables are high in magnesium and calcium and help protect against cancer. Olive oil, nuts, and dark chocolate can help to prevent heart disease. Build your diet around foods that protect and strengthen your health.

SHOPPING TIP

Shop the perimeter of the grocery store and steer clear of the aisles, where the packaged foods lurk. And read the labels! Do not buy anything in a cardboard box or plastic bag unless you can recognize and understand all the ingredients. Always look at serving size when considering the amount of sugar, carbohydrates, sodium, and fat. Read all the ingredients. In general, the more ingredients, the less healthy the product.

21. Create a More Colorful Rainbow On Your Plate.

Not all fruits and vegetables are created equally, and their benefits (or lack thereof) can vary. Take a salad, for example. For some people, a "green" salad is nothing more than iceberg lettuce submerged in a high-fat, creamy dressing. Some salads have 50 grams of fat in the dressing and are made with GMO oils—there is nothing healthy about that. Think of the colors of the rainbow for a better way to get your fruits and vegetables:

- Look for those with deeper or more intense color, such as purple grapes and dark greens. They are better for you.

- Build side dishes around dark green, leafy vegetables like kale and spinach, broccoli, deep red beets, green and yellow summer squash, and sweet potatoes.

- Choose sweet potatoes with a deep orange color. These are much higher in beta-carotene.

- Serve colorful fruits for dessert: strawberries, blackberries, blueberries, raspberries, and pomegranate are all packed with natural, health-promoting chemicals called phytonutrients.

22. Fight Disease with Phytonutrients.

Why the emphasis on color in our food? Deep, rich color is a good sign that a fruit or vegetable is high in natural phytonutrients. The word *phyto* originated from the Greek word meaning "plant." Phytonutrients have antioxidant effects on the body, meaning that they help protect cells against damage caused by harmful toxins such as air pollution and tobacco smoke. These toxins can create harmful free-radical molecules, which contribute to illnesses such as heart disease, cancer, and Alzheimer's disease.

There are more than 10,000 phytonutrients, and they help fight disease naturally by boosting the immune system and providing anti-inflammatory properties. They are even antiviral and antibacterial. Some phytonutrients act like antibiotics in the body and help fight infection. Phytonutrients may have an even greater beneficial effect on our health than vitamins, minerals, and micronutrients.

Whole grains, legumes, olive oil, and nuts are rich in phytonutrients. Wonderfully, so is dark chocolate! Look for a variety that contains at least 70 percent cacao, which has been found to lower blood pressure and raise levels of "good" HDL cholesterol. Chocolate is high in calories, however, so eat it in moderation—otherwise, the extra calories will outweigh the benefits. Dark chocolate can also cause extra heart beats, or arrhythmia, so please avoid it if you have this health challenge.

23. Take a Page from Grandma's Cookbook— The Mediterranean Diet.

I was raised in Brooklyn by my paternal grandmother, who came from Calabria, Italy. She brought many traditions with her to America. Our whole family would sit down together for meals, and she would prepare most everything from scratch. There were few packaged foods in our home but plenty of green vegetables such as escarole and broccoli. My grandmother always had a gallon of olive oil on hand for cooking. The can was so heavy, I couldn't pick it up! She was always sautéing garlic and using rosemary. Her pantry was full of basil, fresh tomatoes, and vegetables. Yes, we had pasta, but it was typically served as a side dish along with much bigger servings of vegetables.

My mother's mother, who came from the southern Italian city of Naples, grew her own vegetables in her backyard garden. Grandma Filomena even made wine in her basement.

What my grandmothers brought with them to America is what we now call a Mediterranean diet, one of the most researched and healthiest diets around. It is based on the dietary patterns of people living in the olive-growing regions of the Mediterranean in the 1950s and '60s, before the introduction of fast food. The Mediterranean diet is not one specific diet plan; it is a simple, back-to-basics way of eating that promotes the use of monounsaturated fat such as olive oil and certain types of nuts. It emphasizes vegetables, fruits, and whole grains.

It's never too late to incorporate the best principles of this diet into your life. In fact, the HALE Trial Project of 2004 studied individuals aged 70 to 90 who followed a Mediterranean-style diet, walked daily, and quit smoking. Their rate of cardiac events and mortality dropped by more than 50 percent.

Today, I recommend that my patients, especially those with documented coronary or vascular disease, eat an even stricter low-fat, vegetarian diet for plaque reversal. We know now from years of studies and from the results of Dr. Dean Ornish's Lifestyle Change Program that a vegetarian diet of 10 percent fat can reverse plaque in blood vessels and decrease chest pain symptoms by 91 percent. In 2013, the PREDIMED study demonstrated a 30 percent reduction in cardiovascular events in those individuals eating a Mediterranean diet supplemented with extra-virgin olive oil or nuts.

How does your diet measure up? Take the 14-point Mediterranean Diet Test in Appendix C.

Mediterranean Diet May Be Better Than Medication, Study Finds

The Lyon Diet Heart Study was a very large, five-year trial that studied the effects of a Mediterranean diet on people with documented coronary artery disease. Because the results were so impressive, researchers actually concluded the study ahead of schedule. Study participants had a 70 percent reduction in cardiovascular events. There is not a drug on the market that can give us a 50 to 70 percent reduction in morbidity and mortality. What's even more astounding? The study found that the likelihood of developing cancer later in life dropped by 80 percent.

24. Eat More Good Fats and Less Bad Fats.

Fat sometimes gets a bad rap. Dietary fat is one of the three macronutrients—along with protein and carbohydrates—that give our bodies energy and support vital functions. Vitamins A and D, for example, are stored in our fat cells. So which fats should you eat, and which ones should you limit or avoid?

— **Saturated fats** are known as "bad" fats because they are linked to serious diseases such as cancer and coronary heart disease. They are solid at room temperature and include animal fats such as those in beef, pork, and lamb as well as butter, cream, and cheese. People who participated in the Lyon Heart Study were asked to avoid saturated fat. You should avoid them, too—along with hydrogenated fats, trans fats, and partially hydrogenated oils. Not surprisingly, common examples with fats from this last group include margarine, biscuits, pastries, and deep-fried fast foods, such as doughnuts and French fries.

— **Unsaturated fats**, or "good" fats, generally come from vegetables, nuts, and fish. They fall into two categories: monounsaturated and polyunsaturated.

- **Monounsaturated fats** can help reduce bad cholesterol levels and lower your risk of heart disease and stroke. In addition, they are good sources of vitamin E. Monounsaturated fats include those in nuts such as almonds, avocados, olives, and olive oil. These fats tend to be liquid at room temperature and begin to solidify when chilled.

- **Polyunsaturated fats** are mostly found in plant-based foods and oils and have been shown to reduce the risk of heart disease by decreasing inflammation. There are two groups of polyunsaturated fats: omega-3s and omega-6s.

- **Omega-3 fatty acids** come from fish such as sockeye salmon, sardines, mackerel, anchovy, and herring.

- **Omega-6 fatty acids** come from corn oil, safflower oil, sunflower oil, and a few other oils.

It's not that omega-6 is "bad" and omega-3 is "good." The problem is that most Americans eat way too much omega-6 and not nearly enough omega-3. The ideal omega-6 to omega-3 ratio is 2:1. The typical American diet is 20:1 or even 50:1, depending on your specific food choices.

When choosing food sources, remember that sardines and wild salmon are high in omega-3. You can also try omega-3 eggs, which have a better ratio than typical eggs.

Olive oil has an omega-6 to omega-3 ratio of around 13:1. This is one of the best ratios for oil, and I recommend it in small amounts on salads and cooked vegetables. Keep in mind, when cooking, that the low smoke point of olive oil can actually cause oxidation and lead to disease. This is why I recommend using coconut oil or grapeseed oil for cooking.

The perfect oil, with an omega-6 to omega-3 ratio of 1:1, is macadamia nut. (Remember, all oils are high in calories, so use them sparingly.)

A *Smashing* Way to Get Your Omega-3s

Here's an easy way to remember the best sources of omega-3. Think of the word *smash*, which is an acronym for "sardines, mackerel, anchovies, wild salmon, and herring."

You should try to have two servings per week of fish high in omega-3s, or a vegetarian substitute, such as flax, chia, or hemp seeds; or cooked spinach.

25. Go for the "Good" Carbs:
Those with a Low Glycemic Load.

Not all carbohydrates are created equal—bread made from refined white flour affects our body differently from bread made from 100 percent whole grains. Quick-to-digest carbs (most "white" foods, like sugar, pasta, or bread) rapidly increase blood sugar and then cause a rapid crash. Foods with lots of fiber or those that have carbs combined with fat or protein raise blood sugar slowly, providing steadier, healthier energy.

Glycemic index and glycemic load are scientific measurements that allow us to rank foods according to the impact their carbohydrates have on raising our blood sugar and insulin levels. The scale runs from 0 (low glycemic) to 100 (high glycemic). High-glycemic foods can send our blood sugar and insulin levels soaring. These spikes and crashes are not good for our health, energy, or mood. The lower a food is on the scale, the better.

When we eat a whole fruit, such as an apple, the sugar that occurs naturally in it enters our bloodstream. This raises our blood sugar and our insulin level, which is usually bad news for our health. However, because we're eating a *whole* apple, we also get fiber, which slows down the absorption of the sugar and prevents an insulin spike. And the fiber makes us feel fuller. An apple is an example of a low-glycemic fruit.

What if we drink apple juice instead? We get all the sugar and none of the fiber. Because the fiber has been removed, the juice almost pours right into our bloodstream. Our body sees nothing but sugar—lots of it. We get a "sugar rush" for a little while, but then our body produces insulin, and our blood sugar (as well as our energy) level comes crashing down.

Exchange your high-glycemic foods for low-glycemic ones. Instead of drinking fruit juice, have low-sugar fruits such as apples, berries, oranges, peaches, pears, and plums. Remember to eat lots of cruciferous and green leafy vegetables as well; they are very low on the glycemic index and filled with fiber, magnesium, and calcium. Check the chart in Appendix D for other options.

26. Make Fiber Your New Best Friend.

One of the greatest benefits of eating whole foods is the soluble fiber they provide. Ideally, you should get about 35 grams of fiber daily. There are many excellent soluble fiber supplements that you can add to a smoothie; however, it is important to add fiber to your diet gradually to avoid gas and bloating. So please, don't eat 35 grams of fiber at once in the form of a supplement. Not only will you be extremely uncomfortable, but you will also lose the digestive benefits of eating fiber throughout the day.

The following are my top five sources of fiber:

- **Whole grains:** Many whole-grain products contain psyllium, one of the most powerful types of soluble fiber, which has been shown to reduce the risk of coronary heart disease, lower cholesterol, and even lower blood sugar. If you're gluten sensitive, try gluten-free, steel-cut oats, quinoa, and brown rice.

- **Vegetables:** Green leafy vegetables such as arugula, spinach, bok choy, Brussels sprouts, mustard greens, kale, cabbage, collard greens, and watercress are excellent sources of fiber.

   You can eat unlimited amounts of nonstarchy vegetables, including the above, as well as artichokes, asparagus, bamboo shoots, bell peppers, broccoli, cauliflower, okra, onions, Swiss chard, summer squash, and zucchini. These are your nutrition superstars.

- **Fruits:** Eat two to three whole fruits per day. Low-sugar fruits such as apples, cherries, peaches, pears, plums, and berries are all good choices, but make sure to buy them organic. These all have thin skins, which offer little protection from chemical pesticides. Blueberries contain anthocyanosides, some of the most potent antioxidants for your heart, eyes, and brain.

- **Nuts:** Rich in fiber, nuts also provide protein, magnesium, zinc, calcium, and vitamin E. Walnuts have more than 16 polyphenols, which are phytonutrients with strong antioxidant abilities. Nuts make a nutritious garnish for salads, oatmeal, and stir-fry dishes. Be sure to watch your portions, though, because nuts are high in calories. Just 10 walnut halves or 15 to 20 almonds contain about 180 calories.

- **Legumes:** Legumes, which include beans, peas, and lentils, supply a significant amount of fiber and are a great source of vegetable protein.

Shopping Tip: How Do You Know If a Grain Is a Whole Grain?

Look for "100% Whole Grains" on the label. Food labeled as "multigrain" may not be whole grain, so the Whole Grains Council created official packaging symbols to help. The 100% Whole Grain Stamp identifies food that contains whole grain in each labeled serving and certifies that *all* the grain is whole grain. The basic Whole Grain Stamp (which does not include "100%") indicates that the food contains at least half a serving of whole grain per serving size.

27. Fight Inflammation with the Right Foods.

Just as we can avoid foods that trigger inflammation, we can also choose foods that put out existing fire. Food sensitivities are a potent source of inflammation, so you may want to first try the elimination diet to eliminate these triggers.

The following are my top eight anti-inflammatory food choices. (See Chapter 3 for more on inflammatory foods to avoid.)

- **Cruciferous vegetables.** Fill up on kale, broccoli, cauliflower, arugula, watercress, cabbage, and Brussels sprouts. Cruciferous vegetables of all types turn on detoxifying liver enzymes and are high in fiber, calcium, and magnesium. Remember to buy organic especially for the Dirty Dozen foods discussed in Chapter 3.

- **Oily fish high in omega-3 fatty acids.** These include sardines, mackerel, anchovies, wild salmon, and herring. Avoid fish high in mercury, such as swordfish, grouper, and tile. Omega-3 supplements are okay as a substitute for eating fish. For vegetarians, I recommend flax and DHA from algae.

- **Low-glycemic-load foods.** Choose foods with the lowest glycemic index and load. Copy the glycemic index in Appendix D and carry it with you when you shop.

- **Filtered water (not from a plastic bottle).** It should be your main beverage. Avoid soda, fruit juice, and excess alcohol.

- **Tea.** Organic black, tulsi, and green tea have strong anti-inflammatory properties. You can even buy organic green teas that contain tulsi, which is known as holy basil in India. Drink tea throughout the day as a main beverage, second only to water. Saffron tea is another great choice and has been shown to improve depression.

- **Herbs and spices.** When used in generous quantities, they have strong anti-inflammatory effects. Turmeric contains a powerful compound called curcumin; research has shown that turmeric can be as good as hydrocortisone and ibuprofen for reducing inflammation. Ginger, rosemary, cardamom, and basil are also all good choices. Keep basil, rosemary, and mint plants in your kitchen.

- **Coconut oil, grape-seed oil, and organic butter.** These should be among your top choices for cooking and baking. Virgin coconut oil is a medium-chain triglyceride and goes directly to the liver to produce energy. It is also filled with calcium, magnesium, and iodine. Coconut oil is very stable and heat resistant.

- **Organic foods.** Again, buy organic foods whenever possible. Herbicides and pesticides can leave toxic residues that trigger inflammation.

28. Get More Protein from Vegetarian Sources.

If reversing heart disease is your goal, consider going vegetarian. A vegetarian diet is anti-inflammatory, high in fiber, and low in cholesterol.

Some people worry about getting enough protein on a vegetarian diet. After all, every cell in your body contains protein. It helps build and repair bones, muscles, tissues, skin, and blood, and it is used in the production of many enzymes and hormones. But when I became a vegetarian, I discovered that you don't need meat products to nourish your body to thrive. In fact, many nonmeat proteins were even better, including omega-3 eggs, low-fat organic yogurt, organic tofu, tempeh, beans, and lentils.

The following are some of the best vegetarian protein choices:

- **Legumes, such as peas, beans, and lentils.** These are good sources of protein and provide fiber as well. One cup of green peas contains almost 8 grams of protein, while a cup of kidney beans packs about 13 grams. Garbanzo beans, also called chickpeas, contain 7 grams of protein in just half a cup. Organic soybean-based foods are great vegetarian sources of protein.

Tempeh and tofu contain 15 to 20 grams per half cup, and boiled edamame have about 8 grams per half cup. If you buy canned beans, rinse them first to reduce the sodium.

- **Grains.** Most grains contain a small amount of protein. Quinoa, which is really a seed, packs more than 8 grams per cup and all nine essential amino acids that the body needs for growth and repair. This is why quinoa is called a perfect protein. Quinoa vegetable burgers make great meat substitutes.

- **Nuts:** Nuts, especially walnuts and almonds, contain both protein and "good" fats. However, they are high in calories, so use them sparingly. The same is true for nut butters, such as almond butter.

Need an easier way to get more protein? Here's how I do it.

There are many plant-based protein choices such as rice and pea, which are also the most hypoallergenic. Whey protein is also a good vegetarian source. (Note, however, that whey is derived from milk.)

I start my day with a protein smoothie. Or I substitute a bowl of quinoa with walnuts and fruit for a traditional bacon-and-egg breakfast.

I also cook with a slow cooker, which can be set up in the morning before I go to work. I like to make bean stews and chili by adding tomatoes, onions, vegetables, beans, and anti-inflammatory spices such as turmeric. By the time I get home, a hot, healthy meal is waiting.

For lunch, I might toss some beans into a vegetable salad or have a bowl of lentil soup. For dinner, I enjoy vegetable or quinoa burgers, quinoa pasta with marinara sauce, or a tofu and vegetable stir-fry over brown rice.

How to Make a Heart-Healthy Smoothie

Mix unsweetened almond, organic soy, coconut, or rice milk in a blender with fiber (unbleached psyllium, flax, or chia), organic frozen berries and a high-quality protein powder (such as one made from organic pea or rice). If you need extra calories, add almond or peanut butter. Slowly increase the amount of fiber in the recipe as your gut allows.

I recommend a smoothie in the morning and another midday, especially if you get hungry around 3 to 4 P.M. Smoothies are a great way to take your supplements. I add vitamin D, turmeric, and even omega-3 fish oil to mine.

29. Lower Cholesterol Levels with the Right Foods.

Many people with high cholesterol cannot or do not want to take a cholesterol-lowering statin medication. I am one of them. While I understand that statins can reduce the risk of cardiovascular disease, they have many side effects, including hair loss, muscle pain, weakness, and diabetes. Statins can even lower testosterone, CoQ10, and thyroid hormone.

My cholesterol awakening came in 1996. Because I have a strong family history of heart disease, I was curious about my own cholesterol levels. My curiosity was replaced by shock when my total cholesterol came back at 320. Within a week, I became a vegetarian. I forced myself to change my taste buds. Organic fat-free milk and yogurt, beans, lentils, and legumes replaced meat, cheese, and full-fat dairy. I went on a 10 percent fat diet. My total cholesterol dropped from 320 to 99 just from changing my diet.

How can you do it too? Start with your diet.

Cholesterol comes from animals, so the more plant-based diet you eat, the more you will lower your cholesterol. All animal products contain cholesterol, and some have more than others; beef, pork, lamb, shrimp, cream, cheese, and butter contain some of the highest levels.

To lower cholesterol naturally, you need to increase your fiber and eat plant-based protein. Here are some suggestions:

- **Substitute vegetable protein for meat protein.** Instead of chicken, beef, pork, turkey, or lamb, substitute organic tofu, beans, lentils, and quinoa. Lentils and beans have no cholesterol at all. Tofu comes from soybeans, which also have no cholesterol. Other options include seitan, which is a flavored wheat product, and tempeh, which is a textured vegetable protein.

- **Choose seafood carefully.** Shrimp and calamari are very high in cholesterol. Wild sockeye salmon, scallops, and sardines are better choices than other seafood, but they still contain some cholesterol.

- **Know your eggs.** New research shows that eggs do not raise cholesterol. It is best to eat an egg fresh from the chicken or one high in omega-3 fatty acids. To keep fat low, it's also best to boil or poach your eggs. Remember to buy eggs that are certified humane.

- **Try organic, unsweetened fresh coconut.** It's a good cholesterol-free protein choice.

- **Get enough soluble fiber.** Try to increase your fiber to about 35 grams per day, but do it gradually to avoid digestive problems. It's an excellent tool to help lower cholesterol. Remember that whole foods such as steel-cut oats, quinoa, brown rice, and beans are good sources of soluble fiber. Any of many excellent fiber supplements can be easily added to your smoothie.

Did you know that stress hormones raise your cholesterol and blood sugar levels? As we decrease stress hormones, cholesterol, blood pressure and blood sugar all begin to normalize. If you perceive your life as stressful, meditation can help you find your path to inner peace—more on this later.

Don't Let Good Cholesterol Go Bad

"Good" HDL cholesterol can become damaged or oxidized. These high-antioxidant foods help to prevent this:

- **Berries.** Choose gooseberries, black currants, bilberries, blackberries, blueberries, goji berries, strawberries, and cranberries.

- **Vegetables.** Choose artichokes, spinach, arugula, beets, broccoli, Brussels sprouts, peppers, and mushrooms.

- **Fruit.** Choose pomegranates, cherries, oranges, kiwis, pineapples, olives, lemons, and prunes.

- **Beverages.** Choose organic coffee; black, tulsi, or green tea; or an ounce of pomegranate juice with water.

30. Use Dietary Changes to Help Control Your Blood Pressure Naturally.

As I mentioned in Chapter 1, the best way to lower blood pressure is through a healthy diet, regular exercise, and adequate sleep—and to transform your response to stress and tension. Studies confirm that this body-mind-spirit approach works.

To lower blood pressure naturally, consider:

- **Limiting or avoiding alcohol consumption.** Alcohol raises blood pressure and is high in calories. It's especially important to watch what you drink if you are overweight or have high blood pressure, diabetes, or high triglycerides.

- **Cutting the caffeine,** which also raises blood pressure. Limit yourself to 100 milligrams of caffeine a day, or about one cup of regular coffee. Organic green tea is a much better choice, with only 20 milligrams of caffeine. (Remember to look for the

"Fair Trade" label when you make your coffee and tea purchases. Also be sure to buy organic coffee beans, as coffee crops are heavily sprayed with pesticides.)

Half of the population has a gene that lowers their ability to metabolize caffeine. These individuals are at increased risk for high blood pressure and heart disease.

- **Using the best cooking oils.** Replace high omega-6 oils, such as corn oil, safflower oil, and sunflower oil, with extra-virgin olive oil. This can lower your blood pressure by about 8 mmHg. However, do not use olive oil for cooking over high heat. Olive oil has a low smoke point and can burn or become denatured at high temperatures. Use olive oil on your salads or drizzle over cooked vegetables.

- **Adding garlic to your food.** Four cloves of fresh garlic every day can lower your systolic blood pressure by 10 mmHg. You will get the same benefit from 900 milligrams of aged garlic extract.

- **Trying wakame,** or dried seaweed, which can lower systolic blood pressure by 14 mmHg. Do not buy the kind that comes in a bag as a snack—it is covered in salt and partially hydrogenated oils. Eat 3.3 grams of high-quality, dried wakame per day.

- **Making a low-fat smoothie** with 30 grams of hydrolyzed whey protein, which can reduce systolic blood pressure by 11 mmHg. Throw in a handful of spinach or kale for extra nutrition—you won't even taste it.

- **Limiting your sodium** intake to 1,500 milligrams per day. To spice up a meal, I prefer using herbs other than salt, such as turmeric, rosemary, basil, parsley, oregano, mint, and dill. If you need a salty taste, try NoSalt, which contains potassium chloride. But be careful if your potassium is high; speak with your health care provider before using potassium-containing products.

31. Keep Triglycerides Under Control.

Triglycerides are the main form of fat stored in our body. Their job is to store unused energy in the form of calories. Usually we see the triglycerides in the fat on our hips, butt, and abdomen. Think of them as your emergency energy reserves. If we became stranded on a desert island and were forced to go without food for a long period of time, our triglycerides would release this energy to keep us going.

Fortunately, the likelihood of being stranded anywhere without food is quite slim, so we don't need a lot of triglycerides. In fact, triglycerides fight with our good HDL cholesterol for space in our blood. As triglycerides go up, HDL goes down, and vice versa. If we can lower our triglycerides, we raise our good cholesterol.

Diet is a huge factor here. Triglycerides feed on simple sugars and simple carbohydrates. They love cookies, cakes, candy, and ice cream, as well as sugary liquids like fruit juice, soda, and alcohol. Simple carbohydrates such as white bread, rice, cereal, and pastas raise triglycerides, as will starchy, high-carbohydrate vegetables like potatoes and winter squash. Certain medications, like beta-blockers, estrogen, and steroids, can raise your triglycerides.

Along with diet, the most important causes of high triglycerides are excess weight and lack of exercise. Keep triglycerides under control with these eight tips:

- Eat low-glycemic foods.

- Take an omega-3 fish oil supplement. Four grams of fish oil per day will lower triglyceride levels 30 to 45 percent.

- Avoid white foods like rice cakes, cereal, cookies, cakes, ice cream, white rice, popcorn, and potatoes. Choose bread that is 100 percent whole grain.

- Limit liquid calories from soda, fruit juice, and alcohol.

- Steer clear of high-sugar fruits such as watermelon, dates, and raisins. Choose apples, berries, peaches, pears, and plums. Instead of chips, dip baby carrots, celery, broccoli, and cucumbers into your hummus.

- Stay away from the chips, cereal, and energy bars. (Instead of chips, dip baby carrots, celery, broccoli, and cucumbers into your hummus.)

- Eat lots of green, leafy vegetables, whole grains, and healthy protein (seitan, tempeh, organic turkey and chicken, and low-mercury fish like wild salmon).

- Make sure your protein powder is lower in sugar and low in carbohydrate.

32. Portion Out the Perfect Plate.

The perfect meal is more than just *what* you eat. It's also about how *much* you eat. Here's how to divide your plate into healthy portions.

- Visually split your plate in half. Fill one half with something green, such as dark green, leafy vegetables, steamed broccoli, or asparagus. Instead of butter, sprinkle on spices, a little olive oil, or some flavored vinegar.

- Divide the other half of your plate in two. Cover the upper half of that half (one-quarter of your plate) with whole grains such as quinoa, brown rice, or wild rice.

- Fill the remaining quarter of your plate with a low-fat protein, such as wild salmon, sardines, lentils, beans, tempeh, or organic tofu.

- Keep taste in mind. Toss in a handful of walnuts, a slice of avocado, or another good fat. Or sprinkle cinnamon on top of a baked apple or pear for your dessert.

• ● •

CHAPTER 5

Supplements: A Natural Prescription for Good Health?

Every day, patients will come into my office carrying a big bag of vitamins, herbal supplements, or "natural" products that they bought online or at a local health food store. When I ask who suggested these products, the answer is usually someone from their bridge club, their tennis partner, or an article online.

You can buy supplements that claim to treat everything from hair loss to toenail fungus. And many people do. About 52 percent of U.S. adults take some form of dietary supplement, and 30 percent of U.S. children take dietary supplements on a regular basis. The natural products business is a $23 billion industry.

It's a controversial subject. Some people believe that the right supplement can fix anything. Others, including some of my colleagues in cardiology, feel that supplements are totally useless.

I take a middle-of-the-road approach. I believe that vitamins, herbs, and supplements do play an important role in our health. But we must remember that supplements are just that: a supplement to a healthy lifestyle. So before I recommend anything, whether it is a prescription medication or an exotic herb, I consider what my patients are eating and how they are living their lives.

33. Use Supplements to Supplement, Not Replace, a Healthy Diet and Lifestyle.

I believe that supplements are an adjunct to a healthy lifestyle. I frequently recommend supplements to enhance the effect of food, physical activity, and mind-body therapies such as meditation. Vitamins, minerals, herbs, and other supplements can be very valuable when used correctly.

Whether you are currently taking supplements or are interested in starting a supplement program, consult with a health-care provider who is both knowledgeable of and agreeable to natural products and trained in evidence-based supplement use. Start by asking about measuring your nutrient and hormone levels.

Sometimes I order blood tests to see what type of supplementation may or may not be necessary. Today we can measure levels of most nutrients, like antioxidants, omega-3, CoQ10, and vitamin D. With this information in hand, we can then make an informed decision. I typically recommend the following basic tests:

- **Bone density.** An assessment of your bone strength is critical to determining the right supplements for you. Having a baseline bone density is also important for assessing your response to treatment.

- **Coronary-artery calcium score.** Calcium in the coronary arteries is a sign of plaque rupture. In addition to treating your cardiac risk factors such as diabetes, hypertension, dyslipidemia, inflammation, and stress, aged garlic extract and vitamin K2 should be considered to prevent further vessel calcification.

- **Endopat testing.** The endopat test is the best noninvasive test to evaluate the lining of your blood vessels (the endothelium). When the endothelium is not producing proper amounts of nitric oxide, vessels are unable to dilate and plaque is more likely to form. If there is evidence of endothelial dysfunction, supplements such as antioxidants should be considered along with aggressive lifestyle change.

- **Vitamin D.** Low levels of this hormone can lead to depression and symptoms of fibromyalgia. They have also been linked to prostate and breast cancer. Many people are deficient in vitamin D; if you don't know your levels, you should have them checked.

- **Advanced lipid profile.** Once you know you lipid values, such as for oxidized LDL, HDL and HDL2B, and triglycerides, your health-care provider can tailor cholesterol- and triglyceride-lowering supplements to your personal risk.

- **Omega-6/omega-3 ratio.** Knowing your omega-6 and omega-3 levels will help guide the amount of omega-3 you need to take.

- **Inflammatory markers.** At a minimum, your hsCRP, Plac2, and oxidized LDL should be checked. Homocysteine is also an inflammatory marker linked to vascular disease. Elevated homocysteine is treated with B vitamins (B6, B12, folate), trimethylglycine or TMG, and N-acetyl cysteine (NAC). Many anti-inflammatory supplements exist, such as turmeric, boswellia, tulsi, and bromelain, just to name a few.

- **Genetic testing.** MTHFR genetic testing is important in determining how you metabolize folate. Genetic variations in this enzyme are associated with depression, clot formation, and elevated homocysteine. Knowing your MTHFR status helps determine if you need an activated form of folic acid or not. Other genes can also be evaluated to help determine if you require higher doses of vitamin D or supplement support for proper detoxification.

- **Adrenal Stress Index.** This test is one of the most important in my practice. It allows for the determination of levels of cortisol, a critical stress hormone, at 4 to 5 points in time during the day. With this information, important protocols can be put into place for adrenal fatigue and stress.

- **Food sensitivity testing.** Tests may be necessary to guide your elimination of foods that cause you inflammation.

- **Micronutrient testing.** This can help guide you in addressing any vitamin and nutrient deficiencies.

Remember, sometimes too much of a good thing can be a bad thing. It's vital that you take the *right amount* of a supplement to get its benefits. Too much niacin, for example, can cause liver damage, arrhythmia (irregular heartbeats), or gout. Too much B6 is associated with peripheral neuropathy (nerve damage).

Many supplements can be as valuable as prescription medications, but not everybody needs the same things. Which ones may be right for you, and how much of each do you need? Since we are all different, it's crucial to work with a health-care provider who is knowledgeable about supplements. You can contact the Academy of Integrative Health and Medicine (www.AIHM.org) or The Institute for Functional Medicine (www.functionalmedicine.org) to locate a practitioner. Naturopathic doctors have extensive training in natural medicine. You can find a naturopathic doctor at www.naturopathic.org.

34. Know Your Supplements.

You can find thousands of supplements at health food stores and drugstores as well as online. Unfortunately, most supplement labels offer very little good information about quality, safety, or effectiveness.

The supplements industry is now regulated in the United States. This wasn't always the case. In fact, in 1994, Congress passed the Dietary Supplement Health and Education Act (DSHEA), which ruled that products listed as dietary supplements could not claim to diagnose, treat, cure or prevent a disease, and every dietary supplement had to carry a disclaimer to that effect. Furthermore, supplements were not required to undergo the same stringent approval as drugs nor did they require proof of safety or effectiveness.

So it wasn't that long ago that I could have gone to my kitchen and whipped up a product, put a fancy label on it, and sold it as a dietary supplement—without needing to prove that it was safe or that it worked. Scarily, it was discovered that many supplements on the market did not contain what was listed on the label. In fact, some supplements turned out to actually contain pharmaceutical medications. In 2002, an herbal supplement called PC-SPES was found to contain the blood thinner Coumadin and the anti-anxiety drug Xanax.

In 2007, the U.S. Food and Drug Administration announced a rule establishing regulations to require current good manufacturing practices (cGMP) for dietary supplements. The rule ensures that dietary supplements are produced in a consistent and quality manner, do not contain contaminants or impurities (no added heavy metals, sawdust, or prescription medications, for example), and are accurately labeled (the product contains what is stated on the label). Later in 2007, the FDA mandated that problematic products must be reported to them within 15 days. Every supplement label must include information about who makes it and where reports should be sent. As a result, many supplements, including PC-SPES, disappeared.

The United States Pharmacopeia (USP) label, like the GMP label, implies that the identity, strength, purity, and quality of the supplement have been evaluated. USP products are produced to what we call pharmaceutical grade, a very high-quality level.

The National Science Foundation (NSF), another independent certification group, also certifies the content in natural supplements. For extra assurance, look for their certification mark on the label of any supplement you're considering.

Before You Take a New Supplement

- **Find a health-care provider trained in supplement use** and discuss your need for supplements with him or her.

- **Check the FDA website** to be certain a supplement has not been recalled.

- **Look for the USP or NSF International seal** on the supplement bottle.

- **Know where your supplement was made.** Each label should have a list of ingredients and contact information for the manufacturer.

- **Make sure that you take the exact supplement studied** if you do decide to take a supplement tested by a reputable source.

- **Take supplements targeted for what you need,** such as bone, heart, gut, or brain health.

Has Your Supplement Been Quality Tested?

Several companies perform independent testing of GMP guidelines, and they serve as good sources of information and quality reviews. Here are a few:

- **ConsumerLab.com** does both voluntary and nonvoluntary independent testing of GMP guidelines for dietary supplements. They put their seal (CL) on approved supplements.

- **Naturaldatabase.com** provides information on supplements, interactions with other drugs, and more.

- **Dietary-supplements.info.nih.gov** is the website for the National Institutes of Health (NIH) office of natural supplements.

If you believe a product has caused a problem for you, report it on the FDA website www.safetyreporting.hhs.gov or call toll-free (1-800-FDA-1088).

35. Probiotics to the Rescue.

I have yet to meet anyone who hasn't taken antibiotics at least once. When used appropriately, they are wonderful drugs—except for one thing. While antibiotics can do a great job of killing off the "bad" bacteria that cause infection, they also wipe out the "good" bacteria that keep your gut and intestinal tract working and feeling good. When the healthy bacteria that normally keep our flora in balance are gone, this often leads to gas, bloating, constipation, diarrhea, and yeast infections.

For some people, even one course of antibiotics can change the bowel flora so much that *Clostridium (C.) difficile,* which is a pathogen, begins to grow. *C. difficile* will cause the worst diarrhea imaginable and requires immediate medical attention. Here's where probiotics come to the rescue! These living organisms help replace healthy bacteria in the body. Probiotics can protect against *C. difficile* and are now given routinely to individuals taking antibiotics.

You've probably heard of a few probiotic strains, such as acidophilus and lactobacillus. Before their benefits became widely known, they were found mainly in yogurt and sold at health food stores. During the past five years, however, they've gone mainstream. Not only are they sold in pill and liquid form in most drugstores, but you can also find them added to many foods as well.

Do they really work? Consider the research. One of the most serious inflammatory bowel diseases is ulcerative colitis, a wretched disease that causes severe nausea, gas, bloating, and diarrhea. Some people with this condition can have 100 bowel movements a day. To make matters worse, diarrhea drains the body of fluid, which can lead to dehydration and a loss of vital nutrients, including potassium and magnesium. Ulcerative colitis can make life miserable and is a risk factor for colon cancer.

Researchers decided to see if giving probiotic supplements to people with ulcerative colitis had any benefit. They gave the research participants six grams a day of VSL#3, a probiotic that has eight different strains of good bacteria. One year later, 85 percent of the study participants taking the VSL#3 were in remission versus only 6 percent of participants who had received a placebo.

This is powerful medicine. If you have active ulcerative colitis, talk to your health-care provider about taking a probiotic. And remember, don't take just any probiotic. Use the specific product studied, because that is the one proven to work.

Probiotics also proved effective in treating gastroenteritis, or inflammation of the gastrointestinal tract. Many children (and plenty of adults) get exposed to a virus called rotavirus, which can cause diarrhea; studies show that probiotics significantly reduce symptoms. Researchers also have concluded that probiotics given during a course of antibiotics have the potential to decrease illness, health-care costs, and mortality.

Remember, not all probiotics are created equal. Some probiotic products contain a single strain, while others have many. If one strain does not work, perhaps you need a different one. Work with a health-care practitioner who understands probiotics and their use. And remember, probiotics need to be rotated after a few months for you to maintain a healthy microbiome.

36. Consider These Supplements to Help Lower Cholesterol.

For many people, a healthy diet—particularly a low-fat, vegetarian diet—will lower their cholesterol. When diet alone isn't enough, I recommend the following supplements:

- **Fiber** can lower cholesterol by as much as 50 points. Your goal should be to get 35 grams a day. When you can't get that in the foods you eat, consider a supplement.

  Add fiber to your diet slowly to avoid gas and bloating. I suggest to my patients that they add fiber to their morning smoothie. Chia, flax, and unbleached psyllium are just a few of the many good options. Fiber will not only help lower cholesterol and blood sugar but also help keep you feeling full for three to four hours.

- **Artichoke extract** can lower LDL by 15 percent when taken in a 500-milligram tablet three times a day. (A few small studies have shown varying results.)

- **Plant sterols** can decrease your LDL by about 10 percent when you take approximately 2 grams daily.

- **EGCG (the active ingredient of green tea)** can lower your LDL by 13 percent. You can take 500 milligrams of EGCG twice a day, or drink about 60 to 100 ounces a day of organic green tea to get the same effect.

- **Berberine** can lower both cholesterol and blood sugar levels when 500 milligrams is taken twice daily. It is believed to be as potent as fenofibrate, a common triglyceride-lowering medication.

- **Red yeast rice** can lower cholesterol by 42 percent. The recommended dose is 2,400 milligrams daily, divided into two doses. If you can't take statins because of muscle or joint aches, be aware that red yeast rice may have the same side effects. Statins can also interfere with coenzyme Q10 (CoQ10) production, which is needed for cellular energy. I recommend taking at least 100 milligrams of CoQ10 or ubiquinol (an electron-rich form of CoQ10) per day with your red yeast rice or statin therapy. Many labs can now measure your CoQ10 level.

- **Berberine** can lower both cholesterol and blood sugar levels when 500 milligrams is taken twice daily. It is believed to be as potent as fenofibrate, a common triglyceride-lowering medication.

- **Vitamin K2** (menaquinone) is the most important vitamin K for bone and cardiovascular health. (Low levels of vitamin K are linked to osteoporosis, bone fractures, and calcification of arteries.) In the Dutch Rotterdam Study, individuals with the highest third of vitamin K2 intake had a 57 percent lower risk of dying from heart disease.

- **Pantothenic acid** can lower cholesterol by as much as 36 percent when taken in 300-milligram doses three times a day.

- **Niacin** can lower LDL cholesterol by 11 percent. It can also lower triglycerides—and raise good HDL cholesterol—by more than 50 percent when you take 2,000 milligrams per day. Do not take niacin without your health-care provider's guidance. Your liver function needs to be monitored while you're taking niacin, and you should not take niacin if you have a history of intestinal ulcers, gout, or liver disease.

Label Watch: Know Your Niacin

Niacin labeling can be confusing. Some products that are labeled as niacin contain niacinamide, which is different from nicotinic acid. Niacinamide has been shown to prevent skin cancer, while nicotinic acid exerts its effect on triglycerides and HDL. In some people, nicotinic acid also causes side effects such as flushing in the face and body, itching, and heat. This "niacin flush" usually lasts about 30 minutes and can be lessened by taking niacin with quercetin or food. Niacin labeled "no flush" does not contain nicotinic acid, so it won't cause these side effects— but it also will have no effect on triglycerides, HDL, or LDL.

Like all supplements, niacin should be used under the guidance of your health-care practitioner. While niacin has many therapeutic benefits, it also can increase episodes of gout, worsen ulcer disease, and cause liver damage. Measure the impact with a simple blood test such as an advanced cholesterol panel before and after starting niacin, and have your liver function checked as well.

37. High Blood Pressure? Discuss These Supplements With Your Physician.

The first step to lowering blood pressure is often a lifestyle change—from limiting sodium and losing weight to reducing stress through meditation and other mind-body techniques—but these supplements can also help.

- **Magnesium** can lower systolic blood pressure by about 5 mmHg and diastolic by about 3 mmHg. The lower your magnesium levels, the higher your blood pressure. Yet 68 percent of U.S. adults get less than the recommended daily allowance. To find out if you are one of them, I recommend an intracellular magnesium test or a red blood cell magnesium test, which can be used as a guide for magnesium replacement. Many physicians measure what is called serum magnesium. This is the level of magnesium in your blood serum—and it is not helpful in determining if you are truly magnesium deficient.

  Magnesium is also good for our bones, heart, and digestive system, and it can help relieve constipation. Individuals with kidney problems or kidney disease should not take magnesium without the guidance of a physician. There are different types of magnesium, each with different levels of absorption. Talk to your physician about what is best for you.

- **Dietary nitrate** in the form of beetroot juice is associated with reductions in blood pressure and improvement in endothelial function.

- **Aged garlic extract** has been shown to slow the progression of vascular calcification and has a mild blood pressure lowering effect. More importantly, it has been shown to improve endothelial function.

- **Vitamin D** can also help to lower blood pressure. We know that people with low levels of magnesium tend to have the highest blood pressure. The same is true of vitamin D. To check yours, ask for a 25-hydroxy vitamin D test. Based on the test results, your physician should determine your supplementation needs, with the goal being a blood serum vitamin D level around 55. Low vitamin D is also linked to prostate and breast cancer.

- **CoQ10** is an enzyme associated with blood pressure. CoQ10 is used by the mitochondria in our cells to make energy. Without CoQ10, we have no energy, and being deficient in it can raise blood pressure.

    Many people start to lose CoQ10 as they get older, usually because of other chronic diseases such as heart disease or diabetes. Prescription statin medications and red yeast rice, used to lower bad cholesterol levels, can also decrease CoQ10 levels. Your doctor can measure your CoQ10 level with a simple blood test, which can determine your need for supplementation.

- **Omega-3 fatty acids (EPA, DHA or fish oil)** are effective in lowering blood pressure as well. Four grams of omega-3 per day can lower blood pressure by 8 mmHg.

• ● •

CHAPTER 6

Turn Your Stress into Strength

If Benjamin Franklin were alive today, he might change one of his most famous quotes to read, "There are only *three* things certain in life: death, taxes, and stress."

There is no escaping stress. According to the American Institute of Stress, an alarming 75 to 90 percent of all visits to health-care providers result from stress-related disorders. When I heard this, I started to keep a list of my patients' complaints: chest pain, high blood pressure, diabetes, irritable bowel syndrome, muscle spasm, insomnia, fatigue, and headaches. Every one of these health challenges is linked to stress.

We are influenced by the world around us from the minute we wake up in the morning to the moment we fall asleep at night. We can't control that. But we can transform the way we perceive, process, and respond to life's difficult challenges. That's what determines the true level of stress in our lives. Our perception of and response to a stressful event is what determines the impact on our physical body.

Think about your own lifestyle. Then ask yourself a few questions:

- Do you exercise on a regular basis, or do you sit at a desk all day?

- Do you get enough sleep? When is the last time you remember waking up feeling fully rested?

- Are you involved in the community, or do you avoid volunteer commitments?

- Are you connected to others in meaningful ways, or are you socially isolated?

- Are you resilient, or do you have a tough time bouncing back from adversity?

- How often do you spend time in nature?

- How do you cope with stress? Do you use food, alcohol, cigarettes, exercise, or prayer?

The way you live your life can make you stronger, or it can make you more vulnerable to stress. If you are willing to change, you can turn stress into strength.

38. Understand the Difference Between a Challenge and Stress.

There is nothing inherently unhealthy about a good challenge. In fact, it can drive you to perform at your peak. But as the number or intensity of the challenges we face increases, it can become more difficult to cope. Enter stress. Then add frustration. Anger. Withdrawal. Our life feels out of control, because we have lost control. There is too much on our plate.

Stress is a physical, mental, and emotional reaction to a situation. Our reaction is based on our perception of an event. We experience stress when there is a mismatch between the perceived demands on us and our perceived ability to cope. In other words, stress happens when we feel like we cannot do what is expected of us.

Think about the lives of new physicians right out of medical school. For years, they studied and sacrificed to achieve the honor of their position. At first, they are thrilled to wear a pager. They are ready to do rounds in a hospital and give 100 percent all day. Their only priority is to care for their patients.

But then life happens. They get married, buy a house, and have children. Student loans come due, and their medical practices become more demanding. As the challenges build up, their work and personal lives start to bear the burden of stress, and they feel overwhelmed and sometimes burned out.

You don't have to be a medical doctor to experience this type of stress. Many of us feel it every day. We decide we have to work longer, try harder, and do whatever it takes to keep up. Inevitably, performance begins to slip. Then, like dominoes, everything else starts to suffer, and before we know it we are exhausted.

39. Know That Stress Will Make You Sick.

Adrenaline can be a very useful thing—especially when you are about to be robbed. It is one of the three main stress hormones that kick in when you are under stress, perceived or real, preparing you to fight or flee. It can literally save your life.

Adrenaline gets us pumped up and energized, and it increases our heart rate. Our blood vessels constrict and our airways dilate, which brings more blood flow to our muscles and more oxygen to our lungs. This is all very important when we need to escape from danger.

The second stress hormone, aldosterone, regulates electrolytes such as sodium and potassium. Aldosterone causes sodium to be reabsorbed into the blood—which may not sound so good if you have high blood pressure, but it can actually save your life in an emergency. For example, if you're in an accident and bleeding badly, your blood pressure will drop from loss of blood. Aldosterone kicks in, pulling sodium from your body into your blood to raise your blood pressure, while adrenaline constricts your blood vessels to stop the bleeding.

The third stress hormone, cortisol, helps control the release of sugar into your bloodstream when you're under stress, because your muscles need sugar to work. Cortisol trades off with another hormone called DHEA. This is our happy hormone. When cortisol goes up, DHEA goes down.

Adrenaline, aldosterone, and cortisol are intended to be triggered in emergency situations that come upon us suddenly and, hopefully, go away just as quickly. Here's the problem: if we feel like we are constantly under stress, these hormones are continually being released into the bloodstream, and they end up doing more harm than good.

Long-Term Effects of Short-Term Stress

High cortisol levels (and low DHEA levels) are associated with accelerated aging, impaired memory and learning ability, weight gain, muscle loss, and even osteoporosis.

In the month following September 11, 2001, the number of heart attack patients treated at a hospital four miles from the World Trade Center increased by 35 percent. In the predawn hours of January 17, 1994, the magnitude 6.7 Northridge earthquake rocked Southern California. The Los Angeles County coroner reported five times more cardiovascular disease–related sudden deaths on the day of the quake.

When I was a young resident, I volunteered to work in the emergency room any night of the week—except Monday. Why? Monday nights would bring a stream of patients into the emergency room with chest pain, heart failure, and other complaints. I never connected it with Monday Night Football until I started to understand the impact of stress.

Acute stress—brief or limited stressful episodes that do not go on long term—can have devastating consequences. Stress triggers more than 1,400 chemical reactions in the body, and these lead to measurable physical changes. Blood sugar rises and provides fuel for our muscles. To increase cardiac output, blood pressure and heart rate increase, breathing gets faster, and we become more alert. In addition, our blood gets stickier and more prone to clotting. These life-saving reactions can also make us sick and, in the long run, threaten our lives.

Make a list of your physical and mental responses to stress. Does your blood pressure rise? Do you develop an upset stomach or other gastrointestinal problems? Are you more likely to have a migraine or tension headache? Do you notice muscle spasms or eyelid twitches? If you have diabetes, do you notice a spike in your blood sugar levels? Do you have trouble sleeping or find yourself sleeping too much? Are you more likely to lose your temper and say things you later regret? Do you experience a loss of focus and mental clarity or low self-esteem? Do you feel tired and on edge? Your increased awareness of your symptoms will help you to better manage stress and alleviate its negative physical, emotional, and mental reactions.

40. Know That Stress Will Age You.

You've seen the before-and-after pictures of Presidents Clinton, Bush, and Obama. It's as if these men went gray overnight. They exhibit the wear and tear of their jobs like a badge of honor. But when someone seems to have aged 10 years in a matter of months, that's accelerated aging. It happens quickly, usually as a result of stress, illness, or both.

In a groundbreaking 2005 study, biologist Elizabeth H. Blackburn, Ph.D., discovered that chronic stress speeds up the aging rate of cells. Women with the highest levels of perceived stress, they found, had cells that had aged 10 years beyond their biological age. The research also linked stress with the development of chronic disease. Stress is a known risk factor for diseases ranging from high blood pressure and heart disease to diabetes and depression.

If a room full of people were exposed to an influenza virus, who would and who wouldn't get the flu? Why do some people get the flu after getting a flu shot, while others do not? We almost always say, "Oh, it must have been a different strain." That could be true. But it is just as likely that they were under so much stress that they could not produce antibodies to protect themselves.

Stress is our immune system's nemesis. Not only do we get sick more easily under stress, we find it more difficult to recover. Janice Kiecolt-Glaser, Ph.D., studied how quickly mild wounds healed in medical students. The students had punch biopsies—little pieces of skin removed—during exam week and again while they were on vacation. It took the medical students, on average, 40 percent longer to heal this simple wound during their high-stress exam week than during their restful vacation time.

How to Slow Down Not-So-Healthy Aging

Health challenges such as heart disease, diabetes, hypertension, and anxiety are all associated with chronic stress. Elevated cortisol, a hormone related to chronic stress, is known to cause osteoporosis, midline weight gain, memory loss, cognitive decline, and decreased skin elasticity—conditions usually associated with aging.

Take the first step toward transforming chronic stress by making a list of ongoing stressors in your life. What steps can you take to improve them? What has to happen, and whose help do you need?

41. Know How Stress Clouds Your Thinking and Creates Havoc in Your Mind, Body, and Spirit.

Alice came to see me, certain she had a brain tumor. A young mother of three in a failing marriage, Alice was convinced her deteriorating memory had a physical cause. "I can't remember what I did yesterday," she said.

Alice had the best of Western medicine at her disposal: a good neurology assessment, a brain MRI, blood work, and even an EEG to rule out seizures. Yet, no answer was found to explain her current condition.

The answer seemed clear after a one-hour interview. Alice was working nights as a hospital clerk, caring for her three children, and struggling with a marriage that was strained due to financial stress. She could not remember the last time she had had a full night's sleep. Alice was on overload, physically depleted, and emotionally exhausted.

The negative effects of stress don't stop with those on our bodies:

- **Stress affects our mental and emotional well-being.** It impedes our mental clarity and makes even simple cognitive processes more difficult. Research shows that stress causes cognitive inhibition, which means we don't necessarily make the best decisions. Have you ever felt stressed and said something you instantly regretted, or snapped at someone for no apparent reason? Stress inhibits our ability to control our thoughts and our actions.

- **Stress affects our ability to relax.** Have you ever felt completely exhausted yet could not sleep? I have done many thorough cardiac workups on patients whose main complaint is being tired or feeling fatigued. Once I've ruled out medical causes like heart problems, thyroid issues, and anemia, we often find out that stress is the culprit.

- **Stress affects our self-esteem.** When we feel overwhelmed and unable to cope, we start to question whether we are smart enough or capable enough to handle our responsibilities—even if we have been handling them just fine for years.

- **Stress affects our ability to cope.** When we perceive that the demands on us are becoming too much to handle, we can get angry. Think of how we describe angry people: "He's a hothead." "Her blood was boiling." Now apply these metaphors to what is happening in our bodies—high blood pressure, racing heart, constricted blood vessels—and you have all the necessary ingredients for a heart attack or stroke. The research on anger is very clear and very disturbing: anger increases the risk of a heart attack by 230 percent.

You may not think of yourself as an angry person (angry people rarely do), but I suggest you ask your spouse or co-workers what they think. If they tell you that yes, actually, you can be a bit on the angry side at times, do something about it for your health's sake. Here's how:

- **Don't say yes when you really mean no.** Adding more onto your plate than you can handle can trigger an angry outburst, even if you're simply answering your child's innocent question.

- **Avoid caffeine.** It can shorten your fuse and make you more prone to say something you will regret.

- **Keep your blood sugar levels stable.** Eat small healthy snacks throughout the day and don't skip meals. Low blood sugar leads to anger and irritability.

- **Get plenty of sleep.**

- **Practice meditation or prayer daily.**

- **Get at least some exercise every day.**

- **Spend time in nature.**

- **Recognize your triggers for anger.** Put a plan into place to neutralize angry outbursts.

42. Tame Your Monkey Mind with a Mantra or Sacred Word.

Here's an analogy for our times. Think about the way a monkey swings from branch to branch in the jungle. Now think about the way your mind races from thought to thought throughout your day—from your regrets and worries to your grocery list and errands. *Call Mom, pick up the kids. Take the car in.* Monkey mind is maddening. And, like monkeys themselves, it's hard to control.

One way to calm your mind is by repeating a mantra. A mantra is a sacred word, chant, or sound that is recited over and over again. In Sanskrit, *mantra* literally means to "free the mind." Some mantras may be a single word, like *shalom* or *amen,* while others may be a string of words, like the Buddhist *Om Mani Padme Hum* or the Vedic *Om Namo Narayani.*

Mantras are designed to keep you in the present moment. They are not necessarily spiritual, although repetitive prayer is part of almost every spiritual tradition. Certain forms of meditation are mantra based. In Transcendental Meditation, a mantra is silently repeated over and over again to place the body in a state of deep relaxation.

Mantras can calm your heart and reduce your stress and anxiety as well. Luciano Bernardi, M.D., studied the effect of mantra repetition on the autonomic nervous system through measurements of heart-rate variability, which is the beat-to-beat variation between heartbeats. Low heart-rate variability is a sign that the autonomic nervous system is less flexible, and it is an independent risk factor for heart attack and sudden death. Dr. Bernardi successfully demonstrated that repetitive prayer and mantra repetition can actually improve heart-rate variability.

Dr. Jill Bormann, a research nurse scientist at VA San Diego Healthcare System, studied the effect of mantra on improving the quality of life in people with post-traumatic stress disorder (PTSD). She found that mantra repetition significantly decreased the anxiety and stress of individuals with PTSD.

How to Choose and Use a Mantra

Mantra repetition can calm your mind, improve your sleep, and decrease your anxiety. Choose a mantra that is meaningful to you (see Appendix E). It will anchor what is most important and allow you to:

- **Be present.** Free your mind from distraction by reciting a chosen mantra while walking, jogging, or waiting in line.

- **Escape negative thoughts.** When you think about something negative, you feel the emotion in the present, regardless of when the actual event took place. Mantras take us out of the emotion and refocus us on the present moment or the Divine.

- **Ease into a state of relaxation.** When you are feeling angry, anxious, upset, or afraid, your mantra will calm you down and allow you to achieve inner peace.

- **Mantra to enhance sleep.** If you have trouble falling asleep or waking from sleep, recite your mantra over and over again. When your thoughts wander, bring your mind back to the mantra. In no time, you will relax and fall asleep again.

43. Keep Your Blood Sugar Up to Reduce Stress and Soothe Your Mood.

I used to work long hours in the clinic, frequently skipping lunch. Apparently, I was not a pleasant person to work with on such days. One day a brave medical assistant remarked, "I think you need something to eat, Dr. Guarneri. I notice when you are hungry, your temper is short."

If your fuse gets short at certain times of the day, it may be a response to low blood sugar. If you find that happening, don't jump-start your energy between meals with simple sugars like doughnuts or candy. These foods cause blood sugar to quickly rise, and your body responds by producing insulin to bring the blood sugar level back down. As your blood sugar level drops, you may feel frustrated, cranky, and irritable.

It's easy enough to correct this problem: stay away from simple sugars and simple carbohydrates and follow these tips:

- Don't skip meals!

- Eat healthy food every two to three hours to keep your blood sugar level stable, neither too high nor too low, and keep your mood on a more even keel.

- Snack on baby carrots, celery sticks, broccoli, nuts, and whole fruits such as apples.

- Make a protein smoothie with a scoop of soluble fiber to ward off midday fatigue.

44. Understand How Stress Affects Your Perception of the World.

Mark Twain understood a lot about human nature and the power of perception. "I have suffered a great many misfortunes, most of which never happened," he said. Yet thoughts about difficult situations, whether they happen or not, can have a negative effect on your health. Uplifting thoughts and emotions, on the other hand, can have a positive effect.

When a group of students in a study watched a movie about Mother Teresa caring for the sick and poor, 92 percent had a measurable positive change in their level of IgA, the protein that protects the body from infection. This strongly suggests that their immune systems were boosted by watching the movie. In the remaining 8 percent or so of the students, IgA levels decreased after watching the movie. The implication of this is extraordinary. We know that scary or violent movies cause us to release stress hormones. How many times have you felt your heart racing in response to an action or horror scene?

One of the most groundbreaking perception studies was conducted by Elizabeth Blackburn, Ph.D., and Elissa Epel, Ph.D., in 2004. The researchers asked a fundamental question: Do perceived stress and length of stress affect cellular markers of aging?

For the study, they chose premenopausal women who had either a healthy or chronically ill child. The research demonstrated that for those women with an ill child, caregiving for a longer time (perceived stress) was associated with shorter telomere length, lower telomerase activity, and greater levels of oxidative stress. (A telomere is part of a chromosome. Telomere length and telomerase enzyme activity are indicators of cellular aging.) In other words, this study demonstrated that perceived stress (part of one's perception of the world), is associated with cell senescence (cell aging) and cell death.

How Do *You* See the World?

If the stock market takes a sudden drop, do you respond with depression and anxiety, or do you see it as an opportunity to purchase stocks at a better price? Try the following simple exercise to see if you are someone who looks at the glass as half empty or half full.

> **Be an observer of your own thoughts.** *Imagine you are an innocent bystander watching your thoughts and behavior as you would watch a movie. Pay attention to how you think, what you judge, and what you criticize. Do you see the good in everything? Do you count your blessings? Or do you focus on what is lacking?*

This exercise is especially helpful during stressful times. Once you become aware of how you perceive things, then you can begin to make changes. After all, we can't magically change every situation that doesn't fit our ideal. But we can change how we react.

Imagine a dad rushing off to work. He's late, and he still has to drop his son off at school. They jump in the car, Dad is driving as fast as he can, and then they get stuck at a train crossing. The lights are flashing, the bells are ringing, and traffic comes to a complete halt. Dad is sitting there, all tense behind the wheel, and little Johnny next to him says excitedly, "Wow, Dad, we get to see a train!" Two individuals may have the same experience but totally different responses.

45. Take a Deep Breath—One Nostril at a Time.

When you are clearly stressed or anxious, has anyone ever said to you, "Stop and take a deep breath"? Breathing exercises have been used for thousands of years as part of the yogic tradition to elicit various physiologic responses. Just stopping for a moment can even make a difference in how you react to a stressful situation.

Pranayama is a Sanskrit word that means "extension of the prana" (*prana* means "breath"). Certain pranayama can energize you, while others help you to sleep and relax. One of the most powerful is alternate nostril breathing (*nadi shodhana*).

Alternate nostril breathing helps to balance the sides of the brain. The technique may take a few minutes to learn, but with simple practice, you will be rewarded with immediate calming effects.

How to perform alternate nostril breathing:

- Cover your right nostril with your right thumb. Let the other fingers of the right hand point to the sky.

- Take a slow, moderately deep breath through your left nostril.

- Next, cover your left nostril with the third and fourth fingers of your right hand. Exhale slowly out of your right nostril.

- Again close the right nostril with your thumb. Breathe in through the left.

- Close your left nostril with your third and fourth fingers. Exhale slowly through the right nostril.

- Continue to repeat this pattern for five minutes. Then switch to the other side.

- Place your left thumb over your left nostril and let your other fingers point to the sky. Breathe in through the right nostril.

- Cover the right nostril with your third and fourth fingers and breathe out through the left. Continue this pattern for five minutes.

- You will almost immediately feel your mind and your body go into a deep state of calm and relaxation.

Practice this technique at least once per day. Use it as often as you need to help elicit a calm state of clarity.

46. Bring Your Hands to Heart Center and Breathe.

Even the simplest breath-work exercises produce instant results. Breathing controls our autonomic nervous system. When we take a deep breath in, our heart rate increases, and when we exhale, our heart rate decreases. However, if we breathe in a cyclical, rhythmical way, our autonomic system stabilizes.

HeartMath is a California-based company that teaches various techniques to transform the stress response. Heart-focused breathing is one of these techniques. To engage in it, the first thing you need to do is to take a time-out. If at all possible, remove yourself from a stressful situation, especially before you say or do something that you may regret. If you can't remove yourself physically, do so emotionally.

Next, get out of your head by dropping your focus down to your heart. Imagine that you are breathing in and out through your heart. This may feel funny at first, but in a few minutes, you'll see that it becomes really easy. This is heart-focused breathing.

Take a full, deep breath for five seconds in and five seconds out. Do this for about five minutes. Next, as you continue to breathe in and out to the count of five, think about the love you feel for someone, such as your baby, grandchild, or pet. Don't just think about your baby, grandchild, or pet; experience the emotions of love and appreciation. Continue this technique of breathing and feeling love or appreciation for 20 minutes.

As soon as you start the breath, you are interrupting the body's stress response, so you should already start to feel more relaxed. You are stopping the stress response in its tracks. If you are having trouble doing this at first, you may want to try placing your right hand over your heart. If it is comfortable, place your left hand over your right hand and then begin to breathe in and out.

Closing your eyes may make this breathing technique easier. With practice, you will be able to do it with your eyes open or closed. Eventually, when you feel stressed out about something (like walking into a business meeting), you will know how to control your autonomic nervous system simply by using your breath—even if your eyes are wide open.

Try heart-focused breathing the next time you have a problem and can't find a solution. As you breathe in and out through your heart, think about something that makes you feel unconditional love or appreciation, like your new grandchild, your pet, or an amazing sunset. While you are breathing in and out through your heart, feel the power of the positive emotion. Then ask your heart, "Give me a better solution to this situation." And I guarantee it— your heart is going to speak.

47. Make Meditation Your Medicine.

When I was the medical director of Scripps Center for Integrative Medicine back in the 1990s, we started a yoga and meditation program that some referred to as "Dr. Guarneri's cult." A lot has certainly changed since then. Today, many people embrace meditation, yoga, and other mind-body practices to reduce stress and restore balance to their lives. I often advise my patients to use these therapies to help lower blood pressure, treat anxiety and depression, and decrease blood sugar and cholesterol levels. Yoga and meditation can even improve surgical outcomes.

Meditation is simply the conscious and sustained use of attention. When you meditate, you focus your attention fully on one thing only, usually your breath or a mantra. It sounds easy, but it takes practice to control your mind over a sustained period of time.

Many people say, "I cannot sit to meditate" or "I don't have time for that." That's how I felt until I learned Transcendental Meditation (TM), which requires only 20 minutes of practice, two times a day, to realize significant health benefits. TM does not require you to change your religion or spiritual belief system. I was raised Catholic and have practiced it for years along with Mindfulness-Based Stress Reduction (MBSR) and Centering Prayer. I recommend finding a teacher at www.tm.org/learn-tm.

Centering Prayer hails from the Christian tradition and has been popularized by Thomas Keating. Centering Prayer also uses a sacred word to place the body in a state of relaxation. Whether you choose Centering Prayer, Mindfulness-Based Stress Reduction, Transcendental Meditation, or a different path, practice, practice, practice. It is the practice that leads to transformation.

You can also practice a simple meditative technique throughout the day. Simply stop what you are doing and take a few focused, deep breaths. If you need a reminder, just put a sticky green dot on the face of your watch or mobile phone. When you see the dot, simply take five long, slow, deep breaths. As you do, focus on your breath and think, *I am breathing in peace, and I am breathing out stress and tension.*

Meditation and Western Medicine: The Paradigm Has Shifted

A study of 127 people with very high, difficult-to-control blood pressure was published in the *Journal of Hypertension* in 1995. Some of the study participants were taught Transcendental Meditation™. They practiced TM, using their mantra, for 20 minutes twice a day, and their systolic blood pressure dropped by

10.7 mmHg. A more recent 2012 study, promoted by the American Medical Association, demonstrated that after five years, those individuals who were taught Transcendental Meditation had a 48 percent risk reduction in heart attack, stroke, and sudden death.

Research also shows that people who learn to meditate have a statistically significant reduction in anxiety and feel less stressed and worried. Meditation has even been shown to decrease insulin resistance and reduce addictive behaviors such as cigarette smoking and alcohol use. Mindfulness-Based Stress Reduction has been shown to increase levels of telomerase, the enzyme that protects us from aging. Perhaps this is the reason that people who truly live a yogic life look years younger than their stated age. I don't know of any cardiac medications that can reduce the risk of stroke, heart attack, and sudden death by 48 percent without negative side effects. To me, meditation is medicine!

Don't be afraid to pick up the phone and find a TM training center or mindfulness class near you. Training in Centering Prayer is available at many churches throughout the world.

48. Explore Walking Meditation.

Walking meditation allows us to meditate during our everyday activities. Many spiritual traditions have walking meditation paths called labyrinths, such as the one located at Chartres Cathedral in France. The practice is frequently referred to as "walking a sacred path."

You simply practice being mindful when you are walking—paying attention to your breath, movements, and other actions. Take a few slow, deep breaths in and out to relax your body; breathe in and out to the count of four. Breathe in, two, three, four and out, two, three, four.

The key to walking meditation is to be aware of your feet connecting with the earth and to coordinate your steps with your breath. Walk more slowly than your normal pace, and keep your eyes gently focused on the ground. As you breathe in and lift your foot, you can say to yourself, "Breathe in, two, three, four." Next, exhale as your heel, ball of your foot, and toes slowly touch the ground. Think, *Breathe out, two, three, four.*

Then inhale as you lift the opposite foot again ("Breathe in . . ."), and exhale as your heel, the ball of your foot, and toes touch the earth ("Breathe out . . .").

If your mind wanders, just bring it back to the present moment. Use your breath as a point of focus, with each breath and step linked in meditative action.

49. Try a Singing Meditation to Find Your True Self.

Kirtan kriya (KEER-tun KREE-a) is a singing movement meditation that originated in the Kundalini yoga tradition. It involves the singing of the sounds *saa taa naa maa* along with finger movements called mudras. (*Sat nam* is a beautiful saying that simply translates to "my true essence.") This lovely chant has been found to increase blood flow to the brain, resulting in improved memory, attention, and cognition, according to a study published in the 2010 *Journal of Alzheimer's Disease.*

Kirtan Kriya

As you practice kirtan kriya, you place your body in the best state for health and healing. Follow these steps to balance body, mind, and spirit:

- Sit in an upright position. Gently close your eyes and imagine the sounds *saa taa naa maa* flowing in through the top of your head and out the middle of your forehead.

- For two minutes, sing *saa taa naa maa* in your normal voice.

- Next, sing for two minutes in a whisper.

- For the next four minutes, sing the sounds silently to yourself.

- Now reverse the order: whisper for two minutes, followed by two minutes of the sounds sung in your normal voice. The total exercise takes 12 minutes.

Don't get hung up on the timing. Do your best. Soon it will become second nature. Remember, practice leads to transformation. I guarantee that your body will be relaxed and at peace way before you even complete the exercise.

When you are comfortable with singing the sounds, add the *mudras*, or hand movements, to each sound as follows:

- On *saa*, touch the index fingers of each hand to your thumbs on the same hand.

- On *taa*, touch your middle fingers to your thumbs.

- On naa, touch your ring fingers to your thumbs.

- On *maa*, touch your little fingers to your thumbs.

50. Make Your Home a Sanctuary for Your Soul.

We frequently head to the spa, beach, or mountains to relax and rejuvenate. What we are seeking is a calming space, because we know it will have a profoundly positive effect on our well-being. Well, what about in our everyday life, in our home, and even at work? You can create a sanctuary for your soul there too.

I once played the "Alleluia" chant by Robert Gass during a lecture, using it to introduce the concept of mantra repetition. I asked the audience to sing the chant along with the artist. A couple of weeks later, I received an e-mail from a woman who had been in the audience. She wanted me to know she had started to play the chant at home instead of listening to television. "The entire energy of my house changed," she wrote. "Even the children are more peaceful."

Is your home quiet and soothing—or is it loud and chaotic? Do you turn on soothing music, or is the television blaring bad news from around the world in the background?

Our nervous system is greatly affected by our surrounding environment. We respond, whether we know it or not, with the production of stress hormones. And as we have discussed, these hormones can make us sick!

My patient Al was a veteran who suffered from PTSD. He wore his army cap to every appointment and insisted that he would eat "whatever he wanted." Al never lost his sense of humor, sharing more than one colorful joke after another. Despite the best medical therapy, though, he showed up at the emergency room on a monthly basis with high blood pressure and heart failure. But why?

Fortunately, Al's wife, Margie, solved the mystery. "Dr. Guarneri," she asked, "do you think it could be the movies Al is watching?" She monitored him daily and noticed a common thread: prior to every ER visit, Al had been watching an intense military movie or sports competition. She explained how Al would scream and yell or become emotionally upset. We had our answer.

As Al became more and more upset, his blood pressure rose higher and higher. The end result was shortness of breath and congestive heart failure (fluid backing up into his lungs). So Margie took over the remote control and decided that Al would watch only the Disney Channel from then on. Once Al stopped watching war movies and sporting events, his ER visits ended. It was as simple as that.

It's so important to transform your home into a sanctuary for your soul. Consider the following tips for doing so:

- **Turn down or turn off background noise.** Blasting television sets and radio talk shows are not exactly conducive to a relaxed state. Think about what you find most soothing, and introduce that into your environment.

- **Do not read e-mail after a certain hour, and definitely not before going to bed.** The light from the computer signals your brain that it is daytime, and your sleep will be disturbed. Plus, you always risk opening an e-mail that contains distressing content, which is guaranteed to spoil a good night's sleep.

- **Introduce the use of essential oils.** Certain scents like lavender, jasmine, and geranium can be extremely soothing. Purchase an aromatherapy diffuser and some good-quality essential oils. Lavender will fill your space with one of nature's most relaxing scents.

- **Create a sacred space in your home.** This may be a whole room or just a corner. I am fortunate enough to have a meditation room. To me, this room is sacred ground. I have an altar covered with representations of deities from many spiritual traditions, and each has a special meaning to me. You can create a space of your own with objects that are meaningful to you. Even a simple blanket spread on the floor can serve as your place for contemplation, meditation, and peace.

- **Bring in nature.** Flowers and plants are not only beautiful; they are very soothing and enhance the serenity of our environment. Place some fresh lavender in the bedroom. Or plant night-blossoming jasmine or gardenias by your bedroom windows and allow the scent to filter into your room at night.

51. Be Resilient to Change. Embrace It with an Open Heart and Mind.

Before stress takes a physical toll, it usually takes an emotional one. When we feel overwhelmed by stress, we often respond with anger, fear, or depression. This can trigger the release of stress hormones, setting off chemical reactions in the body and brain that are intimately linked to numerous health issues, including high blood pressure, irregular heartbeat, chest pain, headaches, muscle tension, irritable bowel syndrome, fatigue, sleep disorders, cognitive problems, and more.

Fortunately, we can learn to shield ourselves against the negative impacts of stress by practicing techniques that enhance resiliency. Have you noticed how two people can experience the same stressful situation, such as getting stuck in traffic or having a major conflict at work, and one will react negatively while the other seems to accept the situation, "find strength in the storm," and bounce back quickly? That's resiliency.

Resiliency can be enhanced by changing your thoughts and by taking action. Here are some simple techniques:

- **Use breath work to neutralize stressful situations.** Whenever you exhale for longer than you inhale, your body goes into a state of relaxation. When you practice breath work, bring your awareness fully to what is happening right at the moment, letting go of thoughts about the past or concerns about the future. Breathe in for four seconds and breathe out for seven seconds. Your body will instantly begin to relax

- **Don't take things personally or try to control everything that happens.** No matter how much we plan, life throws curveballs at everyone. Change the things that you can change. Remember, we can't change others; they have to change themselves.

- **Believe that everything happens for a reason.** Did you ever want a new house or new job that didn't materialize and then realize it was for the best? Resilient people have faith that life plays out the way it should, even when it doesn't seem that way at the time.

- **View change as an opportunity.** Charles Darwin said, "It's not the strongest of the species that survives, nor the most intelligent, but it is actually the one that is most responsive to change." It's perfectly normal to feel disappointed now and again, but teach yourself to bounce back rather than staying mired in negative thoughts and self-deprecation.

- **Build a "tribe."** This is your support network of people whom you can turn to when things don't work out as planned.

- **Practice gratitude.** When you can feel grateful for all the good in your life, the not-so-good seems less important and more manageable.

- **Spend time in nature.** Swim in the ocean or hike in the woods.

- **Learn techniques to enhance resiliency** such as yoga, Tai Chi, and meditation.

- **Tap deeply into your spiritual tradition.** Every spiritual tradition has beliefs and tools to enhance resiliency.

52. Work It Out with Exercise.

Ever notice how great you feel after you work out—and not just because it's over? Exercise prompts your body to release chemicals called endorphins, which work with your brain to stimulate positive feelings. Often called a runner's high, it's that sudden rush of endorphins you get during a run or other vigorous exercise. (Exercising outdoors can help relieve stress even further.)

The positive effects of exercise last even after you've stopped a workout. Not only do positive feelings tend to linger throughout the day but also exercise triggers gene expression.

While most people think exercise is about burning calories, its real goals are to burn fat, build muscle, stimulate the brain, and turn on anti-inflammatory cytokines. For example, the minute you begin to exercise a muscle, it releases interleukin-6 (IL-6). IL-6 increases muscle mass, growth hormone, and testosterone;

it reduces weight and regulates blood sugar. The end result is a reduction in heart attack and stroke risk.

Of course, before beginning any exercise program, consult your personal health-care provider. It is extremely important to ensure that your heart is healthy enough for exercise. While some people may be ready for a rigorous exercise program, others may need to start with walking, swimming, or riding a stationary bike. Starting somewhere, no matter how simple, is better than doing nothing at all. To start, make 20 minutes your goal every day.

If you can do more than that, spend 40 minutes on resistance training followed by 20 minutes of aerobic activity. Remember to always begin your exercise program with warm-up stretching. Start slow and work your way up!

Overall, I suggest setting an eventual goal of 30 minutes of exercise, five to six days per week, including equal amounts of strength training and aerobic exercise. Muscle burns three times as many calories as fat does at rest, so you definitely want to incorporate muscle building into your routine. Building muscle also is key to increasing basal metabolic rate, improving insulin sensitivity, and decreasing the risk of cardiovascular disease, diabetes, obesity, and even dementia. Research has shown that a sedentary lifestyle deactivates anti-inflammatory genes, making muscle an important regulator of gene expression. Remember, resistance training first, followed by aerobics.

- **Resistance Training**: Ideally, resistance training such as weight lifting should be conducted under supervision. You don't need to "bulk up" to see results. The goal is to get your muscles to impact gene expression. I never advise my patients to do heavy lifting (the kind that causes you to grunt). What I recommend is using lighter weights with which you can do a set of 12 repetitions with only moderate exertion. It is best to find a personal trainer who can help you with safety and get you started with a program that works all your muscle groups.

- **Aerobic Activity:** Interval training, i.e., bursts of aerobic activity, is excellent for transforming metabolism. A typical interval training program consists of 20 seconds of brisk aerobic activity followed by 60 seconds of moderate activity. For example, on a stationary bike, bike at full intensity for 20 seconds, followed by moderate intensity for 60 seconds. The goal is to reach 20 minutes of interval training per day. Remember, you must have a cardiovascular evaluation (including a stress test) before embarking on this form of training.

Calculate Your Target Heart Rate

Start with the number 220. Then subtract your age. (For example, if you are 50, subtract 50 from 220.) Now multiply this new number by 0.6 for the lower range (60 percent) of your heart rate, and multiply it by 0.8 for the upper range (80 percent) of your heart rate.

53. Get More Sleep, Feel Less Stressed.

Every day I receive a call from one of my patients requesting a medication or supplement for sleep. Nearly half of Americans don't get enough sleep, yet most aren't doing much about it (besides looking for pills).

When you don't get enough sleep or your sleep is often interrupted, you may experience a rise in your stress hormones such as cortisol and adrenaline. (Alcohol is a common cause of sleep interruption.) This can lead to heart disease, high blood pressure, diabetes, arrhythmia, and depression. Sleep apnea, a condition in which you stop breathing at night, deprives the brain and heart of much-needed oxygen. If your spouse or partner mentions that you snore or stop breathing, ask your health-care provider to test you for sleep apnea. Other signs of sleep apnea include morning headaches, daytime fatigue and sleepiness, unexplained weight gain, mental fog, arrhythmia, and heart palpitations.

Here are some ways to improve your sleep quality:

- **Melatonin** is a hormone responsible for regulating sleep-wake cycles. As we age, our melatonin production decreases. Therefore, increasing natural melatonin can help produce restful sleep. Foods that enhance melatonin production include dark greens like kale and spinach, as well as cherries (especially tart cherries). You can also take 3 to 6 milligrams of melatonin one hour prior to sleep. Sustained-release brands of melatonin are preferred to short-acting varieties and have been shown to be safe in adults.

- **Magnolia** has been used for years in Chinese medicine to decrease anxiety, promote relaxation, and enhance sleep. Take 200 milligrams at bedtime.

- **Passionflower** has many ingredients that relieve stress and anxiety, thereby promoting better sleep. Take 350 milligrams per day to decrease stress or at night to help you sleep.

- **Lemon balm** has also been used for centuries to aid sleep. Take 400 milligrams one hour prior to bedtime.

- **4-amino-3-phenylbutyric acid** crosses the blood-brain barrier and promotes sleep. Take 300 milligrams at night.

- **Foods that contain tryptophan** or are high in magnesium and B6 enhance sleep by increasing production of melatonin. These include chicken, turkey, chickpeas, almonds, pistachio nuts, and halibut.

- **Hops** induce sleep and are being researched for their anticancer and bone-building properties. Take 310 milligrams at bedtime.

- **Chamomile tea** increases the amino acid glycine, which has sedating effects.

- **Mantra and prayer**, recited before going to bed, can help you fall asleep.

- **Essential oils** such as lavender can help you relax and fall asleep.

- **Reduce light and technology at night.** Turn off the television, the computer, and your phone and remove ambient light from your bedroom.

- **The left nostril breathing technique** will help you fall asleep in no time. Lie on your right side and gently close your right nostril. Breathe in and out through the left nostril only. In no time you will fall asleep.

• ● •

CHAPTER 7

Take a Holistic Approach to Mental Health

I first started this chapter with a lot of numbers and statistics. Yet it felt so impersonal every time I read it. The story of depression and other mental health issues is about the way we live our lives and is a reflection of a health-care system that promotes treating symptoms with drugs, often without addressing the underlying cause of physical or mental illness.

The numbers tell an important story, too. One in four adults in America experiences a mental health issue in any given year. One of the most common is depression, affecting nearly 1 in 10 people in the United States in their lifetime.

At some point in their lives, many people wonder, "Am I depressed or just feeling blue?" Symptoms of depression can include feeling sad, hopeless, unmotivated, or simply uninterested in life for more than two weeks. People who are depressed often find it difficult to go about their normal daily activities. They may have trouble going to work or school, caring for their families, or even caring for themselves. (To measure your levels of depression, anxiety, and stress, you can take the DASS questionnaire developed by the University of New South Wales in Australia at www2.psy .unsw.edu.au/dass.)

Depression affects our physical health in profound ways as well. People with depression have a 40 percent higher rate of coronary artery disease and a 60 percent higher death rate. Depressed people who come into the hospital—especially people who already have documented coronary artery disease—are less likely to do well with surgery. Depressed people have more postsurgical complications and five times the risk of death after a first heart attack.

Modern psychiatry uses molecules in the form of medications, such as antidepressants or sedatives, to change the way the brain works. There is less emphasis on the molecules we consume in the foods we eat or the molecules we generate in the form of feel-good hormones when we exercise or meditate.

There is a tendency today to rely on medications to treat mental health as well as physical health. It is my belief that issues of depression, anxiety, and other emotional and mental-health challenges must be addressed holistically: by healing the whole person. We can make brain-healthy lifestyle choices, particularly in the foods we eat and the paths to healing we take, that can help reduce our reliance on prescription drugs.

54. Focus on the Source of Depression. This Is Where Healing Begins.

There's a quick path today from diagnosis to drugs in the treatment of depression and other mental health challenges. It doesn't have to be that way. Antidepressants are widely prescribed for depression, but they aren't always the answer.

Depression is a complex disease with a number of underlying causes. Before you determine the best treatment strategies, you need to understand why you are depressed.

Is it situational, seasonal, or secondary to a nutrient deficiency (such as of vitamin D)? Or perhaps your mental health is being affected by a hormonal change associated with hypothyroidism or postpartum or perimenopausal depression?

Current research has also linked inflammation to depression. It is now accepted that chronic inflammation, whether from gut microorganisms, obesity, or diabetes, can lead to a condition called "the cytokine sickness response," which is characterized by depression. Cytokines are small proteins that help control our response to inflammation. Just carrying extra weight in your midline can increase these inflammatory molecules.

55. Consider Psychiatric Medications Carefully.

You may be able to alleviate symptoms of depression by changing your diet, getting more exercise or sunlight, losing weight, or taking supplements. In some cases, talking to a holistic mental health counselor can also help. Unfortunately, these strategies are not always suggested as the first line of defense. Prescription medications have become the treatment of choice for depression. Drugs such as Paxil and Prozac have become household words.

There is a disturbing trend in modern psychiatry toward what we call *polypharmacy*. This is the practice of prescribing multiple medications for the same diagnosis. An analysis of more than 13,000 psychiatric visits during a 10-year time period found that the frequency with which patients were given two or more psychiatric medications increased from 42 percent to 60 percent. We currently have 1.2 million children on two or more psychiatric medications.

Is there any evidence to support the liberal use of these medications in the majority of the population? Let's look at some research. A 2010 meta-analysis in the *Journal of the American Medical Association* looked at antidepressants and depression. The authors concluded, "The magnitude of benefit of antidepressant medication compared with placebo may be minimal or nonexistent in patients with mild to moderate symptoms."

Patients with more severe depression do seem to benefit from prescription medication. On the other hand, drugs may not be better than placebo for the majority of people with mild to moderate depression.

While I am certainly not against antidepressant medication, especially for people with severe depression, I do believe that treatment is complex and requires more than a pill or two. Other treatment options do exist, such as supplementation, deep-brain magnetic stimulation, and light therapy. If you decide to try an antidepressant medication, have your genetic makeup assessed to determine which medication is right for you. (Check out www .genomind.com for resources in this matter.)

Speak with your health-care provider and family about your concerns regarding depression, anxiety, or other mental health issues. Get the help you need and deserve.

Your Diet and Depression: The Research Is In

These four studies demonstrate that a diet rich in omega-3 fatty acids, whole grains, and low-glycemic fruits and vegetables is associated with a lower rate of depression and bipolar disorder.

The Avon Longitudinal Study assessed the nutritional habits and moods of women at 32 weeks of pregnancy. Researchers concluded that a lower maternal intake of omega-3—in this case, from seafood—was linked to depression.

A second study of 1,046 women between the ages of 23 and 93 found that a diet high in vegetables, fruit, fish, and grains was associated with lower rates of depression and anxiety.

A third study of more than 10,000 adults looked for links between the Mediterranean diet and depression. The Mediterranean diet is high in legumes (e.g., beans and lentils), green leafy vegetables, fruit, and fish; low in saturated fats; and high in good fats like olive oil. Of the 10,094 people followed in the study, there were 480 cases of depression. Those who ate more fruits, nuts, legumes, and monounsaturated fats had lower rates of depression.

Finally, a study published in the *Journal of Affective Disorders* in 2011 identified a link between a high-glycemic diet and depression and bipolar disease. Researchers concluded that women who ate a diet high in simple sugars and simple carbohydrates had a higher incidence of bipolar disorder.

56. Choose Brain-Friendly Foods.

When I evaluate patients who are depressed, I ask them about their lives, especially their relationships, and their diets as well. I typically run blood tests to evaluate their micronutrient, vitamin, and antioxidant levels. I might also order a blood test to measure their omega-6 and omega-3 levels and genetic testing to assess how their body metabolizes and produces important neurotransmitters like dopamine. These all give me clues about the patient's nutritional health and help us identify genetic patterns that can contribute to depression and anxiety.

We also know from numerous studies that nutrition plays a major role in depression. The following foods enhance the production of neurotransmitters, which are powerful brain hormones that help prevent depression and can even enhance the effects of antidepressant medication:

- **Eggs**, which are high in protein, enhance the production of dopamine.
- **Beans and wheat germ** also enhance the production of dopamine.
- **Beets** contain betaine, which is needed in the production of SAM-e, a natural antidepressant.
- **Omega-3 fatty acids**, flaxseed, and pumpkin seed are anti-inflammatory.
- **Organic chicken and turkey** are good sources of tryptophan, which also enhances dopamine production.

57. Consider Natural Treatments for Depression.

If you are not getting enough nutrients in your food to keep your brain happy, you may want to consider supplements. Earlier in the book, we talked about my favorite mineral: magnesium. Well, add another proven benefit to its existing list.

- **Magnesium.** A study that evaluated the link between diet and depression in more than 5,000 people found that the higher the magnesium in the diet, the lower the depression score.

- **Vitamin D.** Low levels of 25-hydroxy vitamin D are significantly associated with a higher depression score. In fact, psychiatric patients are known to have significantly lower levels of vitamin D. It is best to do a simple blood test to measure your level; a good level is between 55 and 80 ng/ml.

- **Folate**, a B vitamin, can be vital in treating depression—with or without antidepressant medications. When activated folate is added to antidepressant medication, people often feel a greater improvement in their mood than with the medication alone. Activated folate comes in many doses, so it is best to discuss dosing with your health-care provider. (Remember to test for MTHFR gene variants as discussed in Chapter 5. Some people become hyper on folate, so it is best to take activated folate only after proper genetic testing.)

Vitamins aren't the only supplements that can help with depression. These are helpful as well:

- **Saint John's wort** is an herb commonly used for mild to moderate depression. Be aware that Saint John's wort can interact with a long list of medications, so consult an integrative, holistic practitioner before starting this supplement.

- **SAM-e**, a chemical that is found naturally in the body, is a potent antidepressant and anti-inflammatory—so potent that it should be taken only under a health practitioner's guidance. The dose has to be increased slowly over time, as it can

produce serious side effects. For example, SAM-e
can create a manic state in some people, so anyone
with bipolar disorder, mania, or a family history
of these conditions should exercise caution when
taking SAM-e.

58. Shed Some Light On Seasonal Depression.

When the days get shorter and the nights get longer, does your mood get darker, too? I know I always feel sadness when we turn back the clock in winter. If lack of sunlight contributes to your feeling down, you may have seasonal affective disorder (SAD). This type of depression occurs at certain times of the year, usually in the winter months, and is more common in the Northern Hemisphere.

SAD can be confusing, especially if you don't understand what is happening to you. John described his mood and energy levels as upbeat during the summer months. Once the dark days of winter in his native Canada set in, he noticed a worrisome shift in his feeling of well-being. By the time he came to see me, he was already taking multiple antidepressants, without improvement. He was hoping I could find a more effective, alternative approach to his depression. The answer was easy: light!

If you feel depressed in the winter, spend most of your daylight hours indoors, or live in an area that does not get a lot of sunlight, light therapy may help. However, check with your physician or ophthalmologist before you begin therapy; if you have an eye condition like macular degeneration or minimal pigmentation in your iris or if you take medications that increase your sensitivity to sunlight, light therapy may not be safe for you.

Your health-care provider can recommend a light therapy box for you and suggest how long to use it. Light therapy boxes are also used for skin conditions such as eczema, but these boxes use UV light. Look for a device that is designed for SAD therapy and emits minimal UV radiation.

No matter what the time of year, try to grab some natural sunlight when you can by taking a walk outdoors. The light exposure can only help your symptoms, and the added bonus of exercise will boost your mood as well.

Light Therapy Boosts Treatment for SAD

In a study of 100 Canadian patients who felt depressed during the winter months, half were treated with Prozac, and half were exposed to light. Those exposed to light were asked to sit in front of a light therapy box for 30 to 60 minutes every morning. Light therapy boxes emit bright light that mimics the effect of natural daylight but with far lower levels of UV radiation than sunlight. The light is believed to relieve SAD symptoms by affecting the brain chemicals related to mood.

While both groups showed equal improvement in their depression symptoms, those receiving the light therapy improved more quickly—on average, within two weeks. The researchers concluded that light therapy is as good as the standard antidepressant approach for SAD, with fewer side effects and much lower overall risk. Light therapy also may be used in conjunction with antidepressants, and doing so may allow patients to lower their dosage of antidepressant medication.

59. Consider Exercise as a Treatment for Depression.

Study after study has proven that exercise is a treatment for depression. It is now known that exercise releases a substance called brain-derived neurotropic factor (BDNF). Low levels of BDNF have been linked to depression and mood disorders. A meta-analysis published in the *Journal of Affective Disorders* in 2016 concluded that physical exercise had a moderate-to-large, significant effect on depression. The researchers went on to recommend exercise as a treatment for depression.

Exercise is guaranteed to change your mood, so find a friend to walk with, go to a dance or exercise class, or join a walking or biking club. Exercising with others holds you accountable, so you are more likely to stick with your commitment. It is also a lot more fun and, as you will see, social connection is a key ingredient to health. (Also see my recommendations for exercise in Chapter 6.)

Consider adopting a dog; this should get you moving! Plus you will meet new friends at the dog park.

If you have a health challenge, such as heart or lung disease, ask your health provider to enroll you in a supervised rehabilitation program. I guaranteed that your health will improve for the better. If you have orthopedic challenges, go to a water aerobics class. Getting is the pool will take all the stress off of your muscles and joints. Even simply walking back and forth in the shallow end is enough activity to make you feel better.

• ● •

CHAPTER 8

Healthy Relationships Matter

I firmly believe that "it takes a village" to nurture and raise a child. That village might be loving parents or grandparents, or perhaps, as was my case, it is a large extended family. The village is also our neighbors, teachers, health providers, spiritual leaders and friends. The village has the power to hurt or to heal.

Most people know instinctively that strong, loving, and meaningful social connections are essential to well-being and happiness. They make us feel good, and they're good for us. Research confirms this.

Our first relationships—those with our parents and family members—have a profound effect on our lives. As we age and expand our network beyond our own family, we add classmates and friends, colleagues, and significant others—all play a role in who we are and who we become—in mind and body.

60. Embrace Your Past to Change Your Future.

"Brain plasticity" refers to the brain's ability to change as a result of stimulation from the environment. A negative environment in childhood—anything from a parent's addiction to neglect or abuse—may likely turn into toxic stress and impact gene expression. While abusive, neglectful relationships can result in a person's anxiety and less tolerance, nurturing, positive relationships teach children how to control their emotions and cope with a reasonable amount of stress. This implies that our early experiences can be biologically embedded in our brains and bodies and can have long-lasting effects on our behavior.

Many years ago, San Diego physician Vincent Felitti, M.D., made an unexpected discovery while directing the weight-loss clinic at Kaiser Permanente. He noticed that many people who developed addictions later in life had had troubled childhoods. This finding became the basis for the Adverse Childhood Events (ACE) Study, which evaluated more than 18,000 people and found that the more trauma a child faced, the higher the risk of major addictive behavior in midlife. Children who witnessed fighting in the home, parents who were physically abusive to each other, parents being incarcerated, or had experienced sexual abuse were more likely to develop addictions to things ranging from food to alcohol to intravenous drugs.

A negative childhood environment can affect your health and behavior for decades to come—if you let it. While it's not easy to come to terms with a traumatic past, it is the first step in changing your future. As we will explore later, acceptance and forgiveness are important keys to moving forward and setting us free.

Your Childhood Affects Your Adult Brain

These eight early childhood experiences can influence your brain plasticity well into adulthood:

- A mother's consumption of alcohol during pregnancy or while nursing

- Drugs (any kind, including prescription) taken by mother or child

- The levels of motor and sensory stimulation that a child gets

- Stress

- The release of sex hormones during puberty

- Healthy or unhealthy attachment to parents and caregivers

- Diet and nutrition

- Social interaction

61. Reexamine the Behaviors You Learned from Your Parents.

Our relationship with our caregivers as we were growing up can have a significant impact on our health, even long after we begin living our own lives.

The Harvard Mastery of Stress Study followed 126 male students for 35 years to evaluate whether or not parental relationships had any effect on disease in midlife. They asked the men to describe their relationship with their parents in one of four ways: Was it very close? Was it warm and friendly? Was it just tolerant? Or was it strained and cold? What the study found was amazing. A full 100 percent of the men who characterized their relationship with their parents as strained had some type of significant health risk 35 years later, such as coronary disease, cancer, high blood pressure, ulcers, or alcohol abuse.

This was in sharp contrast with the men who said their relationship with their parents was warm and close. Their risk of major illness was less than half the other group's—only 47 percent.

From our parents, we learn how to eat and how to take care of our bodies. We learn values and spiritual beliefs. We learn optimism or pessimism. We also learn how to cope when things don't go as planned. If you become angry, detached, or depressed when you experience conflict or disappointment, chances are your parents did, too. If they handled negative situations in a more positive way, you are likely to as well.

Make a list of the characteristics and behaviors that you have and make a note of the behaviors you would like to change. Do you get angry or frustrated when someone does not share your opinion? Do you try to shut down the conversation with your significant other by raising your voice? Do you have a mantra in your head repeating that you are not good enough? Are you fear-based or light-hearted? Do you see the glass half-full or half-empty? Do you trust people? Are you a patient person? Are you nurturing? Are you comfortable hugging someone?

Now think about your caregivers and how you were raised, avoiding judgment if possible. Make another list of characteristics and behaviors that you like(d) or dislike(d) about your caregivers. Whom are you most like? Is it Mom, Dad, or someone in your extended family? What did you learn from this individual? Are those lessons serving you? If there is a learned behavior that you would like to change, work on changing it. Recognizing the behavior and taking ownership of it as a changeable challenge in your life is the first step to transformation. If there are behaviors you admire in others, model them in yourself.

As Gandhi is said to have stated: "Be the change you wish to see in the world."

62. Create a Tribe.

I grew up in one of those families where three generations lived in the same house. My grandmother was in the kitchen, cooking all day for the rest of the family. We always had aunts and cousins and other family members around. These types of extended families are common in Italian households, and I believe that having a "tribe" of family and friends has a profoundly positive effect on health.

One of the best examples of this, and one I still love to relate to my patients, is the study of people living in the small town of Roseto, Pennsylvania, back in the early 1960s. Many Italian immigrants had settled there, and epidemiologists began to notice that the town's people had significantly fewer heart attack deaths than residents of the neighboring town of Bangor. This didn't make sense to the scientists, because the people in Roseto smoked, and they had diabetes and high cholesterol. What was so special about Roseto?

As researchers delved deeper, they found that many of the homes in Roseto housed multiple generations of family, with grandparents, parents, and children all living together. In addition, traditional values and religious beliefs were strong. Families ate meals and attended church together. These "tribes" were close-knit and supportive.

Ultimately, researchers attributed the low incidence of heart attacks to the strengths of the households and community. They called it the Roseto Effect.

Researchers then tracked the two neighboring communities for 50 years. When they compared death certificates for Roseto and Bangor from 1935 to 1985, they found that Roseto residents had had fewer heart attack deaths for the first 30 years, but then the numbers began to rise. In the 1970s, the younger generations had begun to move away and the multigenerational households to break down. As family members moved to different communities, heart attack rates among former Roseto residents became the same as those of the communities in which they now lived. By the mid-1980s, the Roseto Effect was no longer evident.

Swami Satchidananda, a spiritual teacher and the founder of Integral Yoga, said, "The I in illness is Isolation. The W-E in wellness is We." Does research support his claim about social connections and health? You bet it does!

One of my favorite studies was published in *The Journal of the American Medical Association* in 1997. The study still offers a strong argument today for making social connections. Researchers asked 276 healthy volunteers to have the virus that causes the common cold placed in their nose. They then asked the participants about 12 different types of relationships in their lives. Not surprisingly, those with the lowest number of social connections were four times more likely to develop a cold.

More recently, researchers studied the effect of Mindfulness-Based Stress Reduction and supportive group therapy on distressed breast cancer survivors. In comparison to the women receiving care as usual, those in the intervention group maintained their telomere length. Telomere length is associated with longevity and also breast cancer prognosis.

If you don't have a "tribe" to lean on, find a community where you feel socially connected. It doesn't have to be a large group—even a few close friends or confidants can make a big difference in your health. Many of my patients find connection through their spiritual community. Others join clubs like the Rotary, which does great service work. Is there something that catches your attention—perhaps a volunteer agency or a dog club? If you feel shy about joining a new group, remember that most people feel the same way. I encourage you to take a chance.

63. Find Love. It Can Save Your Life.

There is no greater emotion than love. It makes life worth living—and could help you live longer, too. In a study published in *The American Journal of Medicine,* 10,000 men with multiple cardiac risk factors were asked if they felt loved by their wives. Five years later, the men who had responded that their wives showed them love had a 50 percent lower rate of coronary artery disease than those who said their wives didn't.

In another study of more than 9,000 British civil servants, researchers looked at the relationship between unhappy marriages and heart disease over a 12-year period of time. They concluded that unhappy marriages, which often contain a great deal of stress, led to 34 percent more coronary events—regardless of gender and social status.

Why are loving relationships so important to good health? One reason may be that having a close, loving connection with someone provides a confidant, particularly during times of stress. Relationships provide companionship for dinner, travel, or going to the movies. People who are married or have a confidant live longer than those who are unmarried or have no one in whom to confide. We are human beings, and part of the human journey is to to be connected to people and purpose.

Your loving relationships don't have to be limited to individuals. Saint Mother Teresa, for example, loved God. It was her love for God and seeing the divine in every human being that led to her powerful work in caring for the sick and underserved. Her love was for a higher power, and through that love she was able to transform the world.

Others may find pets to be a source of unconditional love. Years ago, I cared for a woman who was isolated and depressed; she had lost her will to live and truly had a broken heart. I prescribed for her an unusual treatment: *adopt a dog*. She took my suggestion to heart and adopted Shadow, an adorable poodle puppy. From that moment on, the dog was always by her side. Every day she walked Shadow and began to make new friends at the park. Slowly, her depression lifted. It was amazing to see how one little puppy could fill her life with so much joy. "I have a reason to live, Dr. Guarneri," she told me. "Shadow keeps me going."

• ● •

CHAPTER 9

Changing Your Thoughts Can Change Your Life

Many ancient cultures believed that thoughts are living forms of energy that remain in consciousness forever. Our thoughts not only effect our well-being but also those around us. Positive thoughts enhance, while negative thoughts can be quite damaging. I firmly believe this to be true.

One of my favorite books is *The Four Agreements* by Don Miguel Ruiz. The first agreement is to "be impeccable with your word." To me, this sage advice means to think before you speak. And when you do speak, make it matter in truth and intention—because, as the ancients believed, the energy and power behind your thoughts and words stay around forever, bringing love or hurt depending on their quality and content.

When we think negative, hurtful thoughts such as hate, anger, jealousy, greed, or envy, we also subject our body, mind, and spirit to the impact of these negative emotions. As we think negative thoughts and experience negative emotions such as anger and hate, our body responds as if it is going to battle, flooding our bloodstream with stress hormones.

Positive thinkers, on the other hand, do not experience these negative effects. In fact, positive thinkers have lower rates of depression, greater resistance to common infection, and a reduced risk of death from cardiovascular disease. I believe that what we think about expands; the more attention we put on a thought or idea, the more likely it is to manifest. Positive thinking improves your ability to cope with stressful situations, which in turn reduces the negative impact that stress hormones have on your health. In short, positive thinking will change your life.

In Anita Moorjani's powerful book, *Dying to Be Me*, she enlightens us on what it is like to be truly awake and to exist as pure consciousness. After waking up from a coma and spontaneously going into remission from stage IV (four) lymphoma, Anita realized during her near-death experience that her fear of cancer was part of what had caused her illness in the first place. She describes how, prior to her cancer diagnosis, she had been doing everything possible to prevent cancer, eating specific health foods and reading about how to prevent the condition. During her near-death experience, she realized how her fear, worry, and self-deprecation had contributed to her illness and how self-love was the answer to healing. When she awoke from the coma, she realized that she was totally cured, even though it was clear that her physical body needed time to catch up with this realization.

Our thoughts and beliefs are powerful. Some of the most intriguing research on the power of the mind-body connection is in the area of placebo. The word *placebo* describes any form of treatment where people are led to believe that they are experiencing a beneficial procedure or receiving a curative agent while in reality, they are given something that has no known healing properties.

A very interesting study was published in the *Journal of Affective Disorders* to evaluate the impact of the psychotherapist in treating patients with depression. One group of individuals received a placebo and a second group received an active drug, but what made the difference in outcomes was the therapist. The placebo was given by empathetic caring therapists while the active drug was prescribed by therapists that were less caring. The placebo in the hands of an empathetic, caring physician was more successful than pharmaceutical therapy in the hands of a less empathetic provider.

64. Banish Negative Thoughts.

Once, when traveling to a lecture, I stayed at a beautiful Wisconsin resort tucked away in a forest. It was winter, and fresh snow was falling, coating the branches with a soft, white blanket. Imagine looking out of a large picture window and seeing trees covered in fresh, white snow and snowflakes dropping to whiten the earth as well. But as I gazed out of the window, I did not see the beauty at all. Instead, I visualized a closed airport and difficulty getting back to San Diego. I thought, *Oh, no, not a snowstorm! I am going to be stuck in Wisconsin.*

As I stood there, steeped in negative thoughts and watching the snow fall, a young woman walked by with her boyfriend. She also stopped to look out of the window at the same scene that was causing me such angst and marveled, "Wow, isn't this beautiful?"

Her words instantly snapped me back to reality. Clearly, I needed to change my thinking. While my body was producing stress hormones, her body was producing the hormone of love.

Most of our thoughts are based in one of two emotions: love or fear. Positive thoughts like compassion, empathy, and joy are extensions of the emotion of love, while negative thoughts such as anger and hate come from fear. My reaction was fear based: *How will I get home? Who will take care of my patients?* Stop and learn to listen to the "tapes" you play in your mind and become aware of your negative thoughts. You might even want to keep a small notebook handy and write down when you have negative thoughts and what triggers them. Each time you have a negative thought, take a time-out. Ask yourself: "What am I afraid of? Is there a way I can change my reaction?" Your answers may surprise you.

In addition, quietly pay attention to who your friends are. Do you hang out with the complainers at work? Do you get together with your friends and focus on the negative aspects of people, politics, and situations? My grandmother used to say, "Show me who your friends are, and I will show you who you are."

It's natural to vent on occasion when we are frustrated or sad. Usually, this helps us feel better. But if we dwell on it or invite others to add to our woe, we are making it worse instead of better. Make it a point to associate with people who do not reinforce your negative thoughts and feelings. You will be surprised at how they influence your thinking.

As we change our thoughts, we change our life. One simple mantra to remember is, "Right thoughts, right deeds, right actions."

65. Say Yes to Yes: Generate Positive Emotions.

I think most people intuitively know that positive thoughts and emotions are good for their health. But it is important to remember that there is a subtle difference between thinking about a positive emotion and actually experiencing it or feeling it. When you think about love, for example, it might make you smile or feel happy in your thoughts at that moment. But *feeling* love can have a stronger physical benefit. Think about your newborn baby, grandchild, or favorite pet. How does the love you have for each of these feel inside your body?

Positive thoughts and emotions allow us to think more clearly, be more creative, solve bigger problems, and even improve our relationships and our performance at work. Rigid thoughts and beliefs do the opposite; they limit our potential.

Researchers at the HeartMath Institute have conducted many interesting studies to explore the relationship between the heart and the brain. They have discovered that the heart is in constant contact with the brain, providing information from the environment. The heart sends signals to the brain, almost like a warning system. The human heart-rate variability pattern (the variation in time between individual heartbeats) is a marker of the autonomic nervous system. When heart-rate variability is low, your risk of heart attack or sudden cardiac death is higher. A low heart-rate variability implies that the autonomic nervous system is not flexible; this pattern is seen in individuals with advanced heart disease or in individuals under stress. When the heart-rate variability pattern is chaotic, the brain registers this information as a threat and immediately signals the autonomic nervous system to release stress hormones.

Here's the good news: heart-rate variability can be improved through a series of simple techniques that not only change your breathing pattern but can change your thought pattern as well. You can experience this right now using a HeartMath tool called heart-focused breath, which I outlined in Pearl 46. When you breathe, you will notice your body shift from a sympathetic, or stimulated, state to a parasympathetic, or relaxed, state. Your heart rate variability pattern will improve and become more organized or coherent. The signals that your heart sends to your brain will tell it that all is well. As a result, you will have greater access to the higher-functioning areas of your brain, resulting in improved memory and decision making, enhanced performance on exams, improved sleep, and decreased pain and anxiety. This simple yet powerful technique can have a profound effect on your physical and emotional well-being.

Here's another simple trick: when your mind migrates to a negative thought, think of something you find beautiful or inspirational, such as your puppy, horse, newborn child, or grandchild. Then, the minute your mind embraces a negative thought, envision a beautiful golden door with a big, golden key at its center. As you turn the golden key, think about that positive thought and feel the emotion of love and appreciation embrace your entire body.

66. Develop an Attitude of Gratitude.

When was the last time you really allowed yourself to stop and feel grateful for something in your life? I don't mean gratitude for a gift someone gives you on your birthday or feeling grateful to your neighbor for watering your plants. I'm talking about the deep, heartfelt gratitude that comes from being aware of and truly appreciating something you probably have been taking for granted, such as waking up healthy every day or waking up in a warm, soft bed in a nice home instead of under a bridge or on a cold street.

In 2002, I traveled with Rauni King, who is my fellow co-founder of the Pacific Pearl La Jolla, to an impoverished area of southern India called Tamil Nadu. Rauni is also the co-founder of the Scripps Center for Integrative Medicine and has a 30-year history of ICU nursing. We were invited to India to help build a medical facility at the request of our friend, Dr. Bud Rickhi. Since that initial visit, with the support of many donors, a 250-bed hospital with 65 full-time physicians has been established: the Sri Narayani Hospital and Research Centre.

There is one moment in particular that defines gratitude for me. I had invited my colleague Liz to visit the hospital during one of our trips. Our foundation, Miraglo, had donated a dialysis center, and we were eager to check on the center's progress. The dialysis center provides treatments 24 hours a day, and since Sri Narayani Hospital provides free care to the underserved, it is always filled with patients. Dialysis is truly a gift of life, since without treatment, death is certain for individuals with severe kidney disease. As we walked toward the dialysis unit, a semi-conscious woman wearing a soiled sari was lying on the floor. In another spot, a man lay unconscious on a stretcher while his wife fanned him with a paper bag. A young man rushed by us, carrying a nearly unconscious child. All the dialysis machines were being used, and these individuals had to wait their turn. Now use your imagination for just a minute to take in the chaos of this moment. I remember Liz looking at me and saying, "I will never complain again. I feel so grateful for all that I have in my life." I know she meant those words with every ounce of her being, as the only thing that separated these individuals from us was our good fortune and the grace of God.

The health benefits of gratitude have actual been studied. Robert Emmons, Ph.D., a researcher at the University of California, conducted studies that found that individuals who practice gratitude are healthier, exercise more, have fewer physical problems, and feel better overall. Grateful people report higher levels of positive emotions, greater life satisfaction, and optimism. Furthermore, according to Dr. Emmons, individuals with a strong disposition toward gratitude have the capacity to be more empathetic and more generous to others.

Start a Gratitude Journal

Write down the things for which you are grateful. It's a great way to bring the good things into focus, shifting your thinking from the negative to the positive. Every night before you go to bed, write down at least five things that you are grateful for in your life. These don't have to be major (although you can certainly feel grateful for the big things, too). You can be grateful that you have a warm bed to sleep in, your ability to see and hear, the health of your family, or even just the ability to hold a pen and write. As we discover more and more for which we can be grateful, our positive feelings begin to grow. This leads to the physiologic benefits of positive thinking and positive emotions.

67. Set Positive Expectations.

Beginning in 1939, coronary artery disease was often treated with a surgical procedure called mammary artery ligation. Basically, the surgeon cut the artery that runs down the chest wall. Medical experts believed that this procedure improved blood flow to the heart, and for years, it was considered routine treatment for heart disease.

Two decades later, an astute physician began to question whether the procedure really improved coronary artery disease. To answer the question, an additional study was conducted in which some patients had the mammary artery ligation procedure performed, while others received a small incision on the chest, but the artery was left alone. In other words, some individuals received what is called a "sham" procedure. The researchers were shocked to find that patients who had received the sham procedure had the same success rates as those whose arteries had actually been cut. The surgeons had to accept the fact that the surgery they had been performing for the last 20 years was no better than a placebo.

As we've seen, a *placebo* is any form of treatment where somone is led to believe that they are experiencing a beneficial procedure or receiving a curative agent while in reality, they receive something that has no known healing properties. In a study conducted by a group of orthopedic surgeons on treatments for knee pain, two groups of patients received an actual surgical intervention while the third received a sham procedure. Again, the results showed that people in the placebo group did as well as the people in the treatment groups; the knee pain improved in all three!

In both of these examples, it is important to note that patients were truly led to believe that they were undergoing surgery. They were placed under anesthesia, an actual incision was made, and they recovered in the hospital. All the steps were identical to those of the real procedure—with the exception of the actual therapeutic intervention. However, all the participants believed they received treatment, and that belief was key.

Of course, in many cases, surgery is absolutely necessary, even lifesaving. But in situations such as these, it is intriguing to see that individuals reported symptom improvement simply because they believed that they were undergoing a corrective operation.

I learned a long time ago that even the way a prescription is handed to patients can affect the way they respond to the medication. When I was younger, I would give a patient a prescription and say, "Why don't we try this medication? Let's see how you do." I subsequently realized that if I believed a prescription really was going to work, I needed to put my energy into it. Now when I hand a patient a prescription, I simply say, "This is going to work."

It happens thousands of times a day in hospitals and physicians' offices all over the world. The act of handing patients a prescription and saying it will make them well sets in motion the patient's own intent to heal. Set positive expectations and intentions along your healing journey. Imagine yourself well, healthy, and healed.

Expectancy and Hope
Are Powerful Medicines

Irving Kirsch, Ph.D., associate director of the Program in Placebo Studies at Harvard Medical School, believes that all responses to placebo are based on expectancy and hope: if we expect good things to happen, they will. Dr. Kirsch analyzed 38 clinical trials involving more than 3,000 depressed patients. He concluded that 75 percent of the antidepressant effect was also obtained by placebo. With such powerful placebo results, we have to question why 114 million antidepressant prescriptions are written each year, especially when many of these drugs have severe side effects (such as suicide).

68. Find an Empathetic Physician.

Jerome Frank is a psychotherapy researcher who set out to answer the question, "What makes people heal?" In his 1961 book, *Persuasion and Healing*, he proposed that healing requires the patient and physician to share the belief that healing can and will occur. He believed that healing requires an emotionally charged setting and a confiding relationship.

But Dr. Frank did not stop there. He added that healing also requires some kind of ritual surrounding the healing event—like the ritual of sham surgery. One of the most powerful healing rituals is the prescription: handing over a piece of paper that is inscribed with the answer to an individual's pain and suffering. Miracles can occur when this ritual occurs in the setting of sacred space—in this case, the exam room or doctor's office. In addition, healing requires hope!

A client of mine, Herb, was a senior corporate executive who had lots of medical problems, including severe heart disease. He was quite famous in La Jolla and held the title "Mr. San Diego." He was one of my favorite patients, and our relationship lasted for years. Herb came to see me for an urgent office visit on his 85th birthday. Recently, he had problems with one of his fingers, and it was very hard for him to write. In fact, he could not straighten out his finger at all. An orthopedic surgeon recommended surgery, and Herb needed a medical clearance. Herb's cardiac condition was complex, and the last thing I wanted was for him to have surgery. I granted Herb his medical clearance, but before he left, I offered him a Healing Touch treatment.

Healing Touch is a biofield technique that is similar to acupuncture, but without the needles. For 20 minutes, Herb and I remained quiet as I performed Healing Touch on his upper arm. Not only was I doing the recommended techniques, but I was sending Herb love and praying for his well-being. Herb left the appointment with a smile. I gave him a big hug, and he walked away with his surgical clearance. Three days later, Herb called and said, "Guess what, Dr. G.? My surgery was cancelled. You cured me."

I will never know what healed Herb's hand—whether it was the Healing Touch treatment, the expectation that his hand would improve, or the hug that I gave him at the end of the appointment. I do not really need to know. All I know is that he never had a problem with that hand again.

I had been seeing Herb for many years, and there is no doubt that we had bonded. I loved him as a human being, and I know that he knew that. The Healing Touch treatment was therapeutic for both of us.

An empathetic patient-physician relationship has multiple beneficial effects on health. Remember the study I referenced earlier, published in the *Journal of Affective Disorders*, which found that a placebo in the hands of an empathetic physician was more successful than pharmaceutical therapy in the hands of a less empathetic provider? Another, similar study evaluated the impact of a physician's empathy on the ability to control patients' diabetes and cholesterol. Physicians were ranked as having high, moderate, or low empathy. No surprises here: those physicians ranked as having the highest empathy had the most success controlling their patients' diabetes and cholesterol.

In 1998 I had the opportunity to meet a true legend in medicine—Dr. Earl Bakken, co-founder of Medtronic Corporation and the inventor of the pacemaker. I had been placing many Medtronic stents in arteries when I learned about Earl's interest in Integrative Medicine. I decided to fly to Oahu, where he and his wife lived, to see the integrative medicine hospital he had created in Waimea.

Earl was bigger than life, a true visionary. He gave me a tour of the North Hawaii Community Hospital, and we talked about health care. The hospital was truly unique, offering an herbal pharmacy, acupuncture, Healing Touch, and massage therapy. Patients' rooms opened onto a courtyard filled with tropical plants.

I asked Earl about his interest in holistic, integrative health; mind-body medicine; and energy medicine. I will never forget the story he told. While developing the pacemaker, Earl noted that the technology worked better in some technicians' hands than others. He concluded that the technology was being affected by the technician's attitude and intention. This realization led him on a quest to understand how we influence the world around us. This is a profound question and one that is a topic of much debate today. There is no doubt in my mind that it has to do with intention and the power of thought.

When choosing your health-care team, interview a few providers and learn about their philosophy and approach to health. Notice how you feel in their presence. Do they listen to your story? Are they authoritative? Are they knowledgeable about things that are important to you, such as nutrition or mind-body medicine? Your choice of provider can have a profound effect on your health and well-being.

69. Believe in Your Inner Physician.

Many years ago, I offered a patient a medication for his diabetes, and he quickly told me that he didn't want it. He feared the medication would "kill" him, even though he knew almost nothing about it. I told him it was one of the best medicines on the market for his condition, and I insisted that he take it. Well, he did, and he had a profound allergic reaction.

I am not certain whether he actually had an allergic reaction to the drug or whether he manifested the reaction by truly believing that he was going to die. I believe it was his own instinct—what I call your inner physician—that clued him in to his own vulnerability. You might call this "gut instinct," and we have all experienced it at some time in our life.

When people truly believe that they will develop an illness or die, this is referred to as *nocebo*. In medicine, a nocebo response refers to harmful, unpleasant, or undesirable effects that are not true side effects or results of the medical intervention that a patient experiences after receiving any medication or treatment. So, a nocebo response is due to the patient's pessimistic beliefs and negative expectations. Unfortunately, nocebo responses also result when a health-care provider informs a patient that they will have a negative outcome, such as a limited time to live.

Research validates the nocebo concept. The Framingham Heart Study, directed by the National Heart Institute, enrolled 5,290 men and women between the ages of 30 and 62. By following these patients over a long period of time, researchers sought to identify factors associated with coronary artery disease. Imagine their surprise when they found that women who believed they were prone to heart disease at the start of the study were almost four times more likely to die as those with similar risk factors who did not share this belief.

The women in the Framingham Heart Study truly believed that they would get heart disease. Could it be that they actually manifested this reality? Is it possible that we create the things in life that mirror our own thoughts and feelings?

Belief is not simply thought. Belief goes much deeper and is much more complex. Belief can best be defined as the certainty that comes from accepting what we think is true in our minds as well as what we feel to be true in our hearts. Belief is at the very core of our being.

Pay attention to your belief systems. Follow your thoughts and see where they lead. When you stumble upon a negative belief, refocus your thinking on a positive outcome and take action to see it through.

70. Practice Positive Affirmations.

Fifteen years ago, at the age of 70, Harry came in for an appointment because he was experiencing shortness of breath. I did a full evaluation, including a coronary angiogram, to look inside his arteries. I told Harry that I thought it would be best if he had a bypass. Harry asked, "Bypass?"

I replied, "Yes, open-heart surgery."

Harry looked at me and said, "Dr. G., I am not having a bypass. I have things to do. I have six bunny rabbits at home that I have to feed, and every Friday, I have to meet my friends to fly my model planes. I am not having a bypass." And then he added, "Dr. G., I do not need a bypass. My heart is fine."

I stepped back a bit. *Eventually*, I thought, *I will talk Harry into this surgery.* So I took his angiogram to what we call Cardiology Conference, and I had the angiogram reviewed by my colleagues. And 20 out of 20 cardiologists in the room agreed that Harry needed a bypass.

So when Harry came back to see me, I said, "Harry, the entire committee, every cardiologist we have, says you need a bypass. And I agree." Again, he disagreed, and again, I could feel his conviction. He was not just saying words; he truly believed he did not need this surgery.

You can guess how this story ends. It is 15 years later, Harry is 85 years old, and he still hasn't had a bypass surgery. He no longer complains of chest pain or shortness of breath.

I am not suggesting that anyone forgo a necessary surgery or defy their physician's wishes. Harry felt he knew what was best for him. He believed it on a very deep level. He continued to affirm,

"I do not need surgery," even though it was clear from a medical standpoint that he did.

An affirmation is a declaration of your belief that something is true. It is not about just saying words; it is about knowing with your mind and believing in your heart what you are saying. In essence, you are feeling this belief with every aspect of your being.

A 2007 study evaluated the effect of affirmations through expressive writing by women who had survived breast cancer. After analyzing the women's essays, researchers concluded that those women whose writing was affirmative and positive experienced fewer negative symptoms and a better health outcome than those who focused on the negative.

I do believe that practicing positive affirmations and feeling the words throughout your being can have a profound effect on your health. Remember, words are energy, and they have power, so choose yours wisely. Pay attention to how you use words, and reframe negative statements whenever possible. Say your affirmation over and over again throughout the day. Whenever you notice a negative thought, replace it with a positive affirmation. For example:

Instead of saying "I am unemployed," say, "I am ready for employment."

Instead of "I am sick," say, "I am healed."

Instead of "I am poor," say, "My life is filled with abundance."

Affirmations can be created to fit your specific need. Here are some powerful affirmations:

- I approve of myself and I love myself.

- I am love.

- My actions create abundance and prosperity.

- I forgive myself for past mistakes.

- All is well.

- I attract abundance and wealth.

- I am healthy in body and mind.

71. Let Imagery Guide You to Better Health.

The mind is a powerful instrument. If you have ever imagined yourself in a more relaxed or pleasant place when faced with a difficult situation, you know exactly what I mean. You can transport your thoughts using guided imagery to help you cope and stay focused. When you use all your senses, your body seems to respond as though what you are imagining is real.

Imagine that you are cutting into a juicy lemon. You inhale the beautiful citrus smell, and as you cut, the juice drips onto the counter. You love lemons and decide to hold the fruit up to your mouth. As you suck on the lemon, you imagine tasting the juice.

As you continue to follow the imagery, it won't be long before you actually taste the lemon.

So what happens if we use the practice of visualization before surgery? Can we tell the body to heal, require less medication, and bleed less? In a word, yes! Diane Tusek, R.N., and her colleagues at the Cleveland Clinic randomly selected patients undergoing elective colon surgery to receive usual preoperative care or usual care plus guided imagery. The guided imagery group listened to tapes for three days before surgery, while in the operating room, and each day during the post-op period. The results were astounding. Patients in the guided imagery group had less anxiety, experienced significantly less post-op pain, and required much less pain medication. Like meditation and mantra repetition, guided imagery is powerful medicine.

Guided imagery audio guides are available for all types of health challenges. They may be specific to treatments such as chemotherapy or radiation, or designed for more general purposes such as stress reduction. At the very least, when you or a loved one is scheduled for surgery, remember to use guided imagery before and after the procedure to decrease anxiety and pain.

Free guided imagery programs are available through the Internet. Check out the guided imagery podcasts from Kaiser Permanente, Loyola University Maryland, Dartmouth College, and the University of Michigan Health System Comprehensive Cancer Center.

Guided imagery programs are available for insomnia, radiation and chemotherapy, nausea, success with surgery, addictions, and just about every other possible health challenge. Find one that is most suitable to your needs, and listen to it twice a day in a relaxed, quiet setting. Don't be surprised if your health challenge improves or your surgery goes more smoothly than expected.

• ● •

CHAPTER 10

Strengthen Your Spirituality

The journey to health usually begins with nutrition and fitness—in short, the physical body. But true health is a cohesive balance of body, mind, emotions, and spirit. As we evolve, we begin to ask much deeper questions: *What is my purpose in life? If I had one year to live, how might I live it?*

Once the door opens, there is no stopping the expansion that follows. The lessons we learn on the spiritual path are the ones that anchor us to what is truly important in life. The rich spiritual lessons are about forgiveness, service, compassion, and gratefulness. These fundamental spiritual principles lead to the recognition that we are all connected in the web of life and that what we do to others, we do to ourselves.

Research reveals a great deal about the relationship between spirituality and health. And while it may seem odd for a cardiologist to be talking about spirituality in medicine, I've found that patients themselves want to spend time discussing spiritual issues. In fact, 82 percent of Americans acknowledge a need for spiritual growth.

People know it is important to get their hearts and souls back on track. My goal has always been to honor and promote my patients' own spirituality and to guide them on a journey of introspection that frequently leads to questions about meaning and purpose. For many, healing cannot begin until they have done their forgiveness work and learn self-compassion and self-love.

72. Discover What Spirituality Means to You.

There are three words that can change your life even more than "I love you." For one patient, those words were, "You have cancer."

A diagnosis of cancer can change your perspective on everything. "I was no longer worried about the faucet that was not working or the grass that was an inch too high," recalls Mary. "Cancer is the best thing that happened in my life. I immediately started to think about what is truly important."

Questions about meaning and purpose in life are fundamental to human existence. They are an integral component of our path to spirituality, and spirituality is an integral component of optimal health. This is why I always ask my patients about their spiritual lives and practices. Do they have a formal meditation practice? Do they pray? Where do they gain strength? Two of the most important questions I ask are, "What is your purpose in life? What is your personal mission and vision?" I ask these questions because they serve as an anchor, something that makes sense about life.

I am respectful of the fact that spirituality holds a unique meaning for each of us. I personally like the definition by Mario Beauregard and Denyse O'Leary, authors of *The Spiritual Brain*, who define spirituality as "any experience that is thought to bring the experiencer into contact with the Divine." I recognize that for others, spirituality is a connection with others, with nature, or with a higher power. Spirituality connects us to something greater than ourselves and helps us make sense of our lives.

There are many ways in which our connection to spirituality can affect both our physical and our emotional health. Spiritual practices such as chanting and prayer can help calm us and make us more patient, caring, and loving. The principles of love, compassion, forgiveness, and service are healing to our body as well as our mind.

For many, spirituality is truly a quest for meaning and wholeness. It is not the same as religion, which includes a community and a philosophy. Spirituality may or may not involve formal religion, but it is almost always included in religious practices.

Whether we want to admit it or not, science cannot answer all the questions. Sir William Osler, a Canadian physician and one of the four founding professors of Johns Hopkins Hospital, said, "The human heart has a hidden want that science cannot supply." For many, that hidden want is fulfilled through spirituality.

What does spirituality mean to you? Does it help you answer the following fundamental questions?

What is my purpose in life?

What do I truly value? Do I value friends, family, success, money? Do I make decisions based on my values?

What is my personal mission and vision?

Who and what do I need to forgive? Do I need to forgive myself?

Can I be more loving? Can I be more tolerant and compassionate?

Can I let go of anger and sarcasm?

Can I live in the moment? Can I surrender the outcome to something greater than myself?

To be whole in mind, body, and spirit is to be on the path to optimal health.

73. Connect with Your Higher Power.

Lillian and George are in their late 90s. They have been together for more than 60 years. They are tall, thin, and agile. They can bend down and pick things up quickly. They have no physical limitations that I can see. They have been vegan their entire lives, and they make a point of telling me that they walk 2.5 miles a day.

If you ask them their secret, they will tell you it is their spirituality. George is a minister. He teaches Bible study, and Lillian has been going to his class every week for six decades. They are connected to their religion, to their community, and to each other.

They are members of the Seventh-Day Adventist community. Through it, they have made many friends and have a very strong social network. A solid support network is a key component of good health. Lillian also feels that "being healthy brings us closer to God." What's more, in keeping with their religious tradition, George and Lillian take a weekly Sabbath and fill their lives with prayer and contemplation.

You don't need to be a Seventh-Day Adventist to benefit from these simple, yet profound spiritual lessons. Research from the Mayo Clinic demonstrates that people with strong religious beliefs have lower blood pressure, are more likely to comply with their medications, eat healthier foods, avoid cigarettes and alcohol, and exercise. They are also more likely to use preventive health services and less likely to abuse drugs. They have less depression and anxiety, are less likely to commit suicide, and are more accepting of death.

I believe that as you advance on the spiritual path, you become more resilient, hopeful, content, and at peace with yourself and your life. Belief in a higher power or a Divine plan could very well be one of the greatest stress reduction tools of all.

74. Develop a Spiritual Practice That Fits Your Life—and It Will Become Your Life.

At the heart of spirituality is our connection to something that gives meaning or purpose to our lives. It could be nature. It could be a higher power. It could be a person.

This connection is always with you, whether you are taking a walk or sitting in prayer or meditation. Be sure to set realistic expectations when developing a regular spiritual practice. You won't be able to sit and meditate for three hours a day if you have never meditated before.

You may want to start with just 20 minutes of prayer, meditation, or contemplation a day. Set up a small space in your home as your sacred space. Consider placing a few objects in your sacred space that have meaning to you. It is very important to set aside the same time every day for your spiritual practice. Try making that time before dawn or before the start of your busy day, if that is possible. If the morning does not work for you, take some time before dinner or bed. Just pick a time and be consistent. After a while, your life itself becomes the practice. You begin to live a life aligned with your purpose and passions.

When you wake in the morning, give thanks to the beauty of a new day. Before you get out of bed, set your intention for how you would like your day to unfold. See yourself having fun with friends and co-workers, having successful meetings, or just feeling energized in general. Walk through your schedule and envision each and every step with your desired outcome. Then sit upright (if possible) with your spine erect and spend 20 minutes in prayer, meditation, or contemplation. The key is to be patient and consistent. Soon you will find you have given yourself a beautiful gift.

75. Think About What Gives Meaning to Your Life.

There is a Cheyenne proverb that says, "When you lose the rhythm of the drumbeat of spirit, you are lost from the peace and rhythm of life."

That is truly important. I see patients every day who have lost the peace and rhythm of life. They come in feeling depressed or experiencing loneliness and hopelessness. I also see patients who have lost their purpose in life or their passions.

I care for many physicians in my practice. One of the hardest things for me is to tell a physician, especially a surgeon, that it may be time to retire. Basically, I am telling these surgeons that their careers as they know them, which are often indistinguishable from what they see as their purpose in life, are over. This can be devastating.

Think about how you define yourself. As a doctor? A lawyer? A schoolteacher? That's *what you do;* not *who you are.*

We are more than what we do for a living. We might be lovers of travel, hiking, and sandy beaches. We might be parents, volunteers, and artists.

I make a point to ask my cardiac fellows, "When you talk to our patients, do you look beyond their charts? Do you know what has been going on in their lives?"

Physicians are so happy to report a patient's cholesterol level and blood pressure, but they forget to mention depression, stress and social isolation, which are equally important and independent risk factors for disease.

Open your own journal and begin answering the following questions:

> *What gives my life meaning and purpose?*
>
> *What makes me feel secure?*
>
> *What am I good at, really good at?*
>
> *How can I use my talents to improve myself, my community, and the planet?*

76. Call Your Spirit Back.

While it's true that optimal physical and mental health starts with proper nutrition and exercise, there are times when we have to take a step back—and call our spirit back—before we can heal.

If you are feeling depressed or hopeless, it may not be the best time to talk about the ABCs of diet and exercise. Although they both can improve depression, if you are not in the right frame of mind, you won't get better. This is often the case with patients after surgery—like George.

George was a strong construction worker who needed a bypass. The surgery was a success and his recovery was quick, but something wasn't right. When I saw George after surgery, he looked the same on the outside, but he was not the same person on the inside. He was completely disconnected from his surroundings and the people who loved him.

We tried everything that Western medicine had to offer to improve George's mood and affect, but nothing changed. It was as if George were disconnected from his emotions. George's wife was frantic to find a way to connect with her husband. Most of the time, he sat quietly without interacting. Antidepressant medications had not improved George's mood or disposition.

I decided to send George for a Healing Touch treatment. (I noted earlier that Healing Touch is an energy-based therapy that uses touch to heal body, mind, and spirit.) I referred George to Rauni King. She placed George into a deep state of relaxation while I whispered into his ear, "George, I need you to call your spirit back." I have no idea why I did this. I just felt that pieces of George's spirit were scattered in all his hospital experiences from the operating room to the ICU.

What I was asking George to do was to reconnect with the things in life most important to him and to let go of the things that were holding him back. I was asking him to reconnect to his passions and put his energies into what he wanted to become. "George, call your spirit back from the operating room. Call it back from the surgeon's office. I need you to do this; I need you to want to live," I said.

During his next appointment, George said, "Dr. Guarneri, of all the things you could have told me, when you told me to call my spirit back, I connected. It was as if I came back into my body."

George's story is not uncommon. When I care for people after surgery, many seem to be shells of their former selves. I may be right next to them, but they are looking at me with an empty stare. They are simply not present.

You don't need to have surgery to feel disconnected from your passion and soul's work. Just about any traumatic event can leave you feeling frightened, depressed, anxious, or less confident.

Take notice of where your energy is going. Are you putting your energy into past events? Are you holding on to a hurt that you need to forgive? Are you worried about the future? Notice where your energy flows, and when it flows to past events, worries about the future, or hurts and disappointments, call your spirit back from each and every event and cut the invisible cords that bind you to them. Call your spirit back!

77. Forgive—for Good—Your Health Depends On It.

A few years ago, I attended a cardiology conference on the Big Island of Hawaii. The room was filled with renowned cardiologists, and the conference was hosted by Dr. Earl Bakken, the true visionary who invented the pacemaker. Dr. Bakken brought a kahuna—a spiritual teacher, healer, and keeper of traditional Hawaiian wisdom—to this very conservative conference. He introduced the kahuna as Aunty Margaret. She had agreed to meet with the cardiologists to offer some words of advice.

I watched in amazement as cardiologist after cardiologist bent down to talk to Aunty Margaret, this maybe three-foot-five bit of a woman, who was sitting in a wheelchair. She was a legend in Hawaii for her spiritual teachings and healings, and she said the same thing every time a new person knelt before her: "Before the sun goes down, forgive." Maybe because we were on the island of Hawaii, she added, "Go in the ocean before the sun goes down, and forgive." Her medicine and message was the same for everyone.

How many times do we say, "I can't believe he did that to me" or "I'm so angry with her"? These statements, and the emotions behind them, make us victims. I remember Stan, a businessman who came to see me for severe coronary artery disease. Stan was in the middle of a large lawsuit. Throughout our appointment he talked about "getting revenge and getting even." I explained to Stan that he was making himself sick; the anger he was harboring was raising his blood pressure and causing chest pain. I explained that he needed to forgive and move on with his life. "Stan," I said, "it is an important point to remember: forgiveness is for you. It is not for the offender. Forgiveness is about taking back your power."

When we forgive, we are no longer a victim in the story of our life, but a hero. Now, we are in control of how we feel. Remember when I said that we can leave pieces of our spirit in traumatic places? Forgiveness is a way to call our power back.

Forgiveness does not involve denying or minimizing the hurt; it is not about accepting unkind behavior. It is not even about forgetting that something painful happened. Forgiveness is not about reconciling with the offender. Forgiveness is about healing ourselves, not about the people who hurt us.

You can hold on to a grudge, which is like eating rat poison and expecting the rat to die, or you can move on and start to heal. It's that simple. When you let go of repressed anger, guilt, and grief, you open the door to optimal well-being. I learned the following forgiveness exercise from my friend Howard Wills, who is a spiritual teacher on Kauai:

> Sit quietly and see the person you need to forgive in your mind's eye. See their face before you. Perhaps that person is you.
>
> Recite these words of forgiveness: "To all people, I forgive you, all of you. Please forgive me, all of you. Let's all forgive ourselves, all of us. Please and thank you. Thank you."
>
> Repeat these words over and over again. Imagine you are looking into the eyes of the person you wish to forgive. You will find that you have the power within you to recover from most any hurt.

Remember, the hardest person to forgive is usually ourselves. We are often more willing to forgive others then to let go of something in our lives that we are not proud of. Be gentle with yourself. Forgiveness sets you free from shame and blame.

The Forgiveness Project

Fred Luskin, Ph.D., conducted a study at Stanford University called the Forgiveness Project. Dr. Luskin's research validates that forgiveness puts us at peace and allows us to take hurtful things less personally. Through his research, he learned that forgivers are more optimistic, less angry, and less stressed. They also have lower blood pressure, less muscle tension, a slower heart rate, fewer illnesses, and fewer chronic conditions.

Forgiveness is truly the essence of emotional and spiritual healing. Forgiveness is the very heart of spiritual counseling, because it is the basis of the recovery of the true self.

78. Pay It Forward in Any Way You Can— and See What Happens.

Several years ago, at a toll booth in Georgia, drivers began a practice of paying for the toll of the car behind them in line. When the state tried to outlaw the practice, drivers protested so strongly that the ban was reversed.

There's always something so heartwarming about a total stranger assisting us in any way. It could be as simple as paying for your toll, allowing you to merge into a crowded lane on the freeway, or holding the door open when your hands are full. Yet, we are still kind of startled and even suspicious of any random act of kindness.

I can recall being in the supermarket checkout line when I realized that I had a $10 coupon that I couldn't use. I noticed that the woman behind me had enough items in her cart to take advantage of the coupon, so I reached over and handed it to her. She looked at me as if I were crazy and then asked, "Will this really work?" Once convinced that I had no hidden agenda, she relaxed, thanked me profusely, smiled, and proceeded to check out.

I didn't expect anything from this woman in return, but perhaps she will do something nice for someone else in the future. True giving is not conditional; it comes from the heart. The joy we bring to others brings joy to us.

It doesn't matter how small the gesture. When you give of yourself and expect nothing in return, the sentiment is always appreciated. So, open the door for someone, help carry a package or suitcase, or pay someone's toll. I can guarantee that they will pay it forward and your heart will be filled with joy.

79. Pray It All Away.

I was raised Catholic and taught that Jesus had the ability to heal, yet I never truly understood spiritual healing. There is mention of healing throughout the New Testament, so much so that my Aunt Gina referred to Jesus as the Divine Physician. Although it was never explicitly stated, I was raised to believe that this power was limited to Jesus and not available to others. This is ironic, since one of Jesus's most famous quotes is: "You shall do what I do and more."

Following the publication of my first book, *The Heart Speaks*, I received a call from Reverend Robert Schuller, founder of the Crystal Cathedral and the weekly television program *Hour of Power*. Dr. Schuller was intrigued by my book and wanted permission to talk about it on *Larry King Live*.

I was invited to lunch at the Crystal Cathedral to meet with Dr. Schuller and his staff. Before lunch I toured the cathedral and was invited to meditate in a room that Dr. Schuller called his "dream room." The room was narrow and very tall—perhaps three stories high—and entirely white. At the front was a huge statue of Jesus. I sat on a chair in the center of the room and marveled at the peace and tranquility I felt.

Twenty minutes later, Dr. Schuller returned and reminded me that it was time for lunch, but he said that first, he wanted to give me some important information. He offered me a spiritual healing, and the next thing I remember is Dr. Schuller placing his right hand over my forehead, covering what mystics would call my third eye. Instantly, I felt as if I were going to faint. My legs began to weaken, and I felt as if I were out of my body. I could feel a stream of energy pouring from Dr. Schuller's hand into the top of my head. To this day I wonder what information Dr. Schuller shared. I am sure my soul knows. All I know is that I had a major spiritual experience—what some would definitely call a healing or a transmission of healing energy. Over lunch Reverend Schuller described the power of prayer: "Prayers are energy. All prayers are heard, and all prayers are answered."

This was not the first or last time I would hear about the power of prayer. I met with spiritual teacher Howard Wills while I was completing this section of the book. One day, he called to say hello; it was the first time we had talked in more than a year. I laughed and said, "Funny you should call when I am writing about spiritual healers."

Howard's instant response was, "Tell everyone, Mimi, to pray it all away, no matter what their problem is. Pray it all away."

Howard's prayers are for forgiveness and the creation of right relationships with ourselves, others, the planet, and our ancestral lineage. "Just like you sweep your house on a daily basis, you need to sweep yourself clean in order to heal and remain healthy," he says. I believe this is wise advice.

The following prayer is shared, with Howard's permission, to cleanse your entire lineage. Say this prayer ten times per day to help heal body, mind, and spirit.

Generational Cleansing Prayer

Infinite Light,
For Me, My Family, And Our Entire Lineage,
And All Humanity
Throughout All Time, Past, Present, And Future.
Please Help Us All Forgive Each Other,
Forgive Ourselves, Forgive All People,
And All People Forgive Us
Completely And Totally, Now And Forever.
Please And Thank You, Thank You.

• ● •

CHAPTER 11

The Energy to Heal

Have you ever walked into a room and immediately felt uncomfortable for no apparent reason? Even if no one was arguing, you could sense that there has just been a fight. Or perhaps you have felt the opposite, such as the peace you might feel walking into a spiritual center. It is as if the room itself is holding the energy or vibration of what has occurred in that space.

In a similar sense, while you may not be able to physically see someone's energy, you certainly can feel and be affected by it. Positive energy invigorates you. Negative energy can drag you down. This feeling is universally understood. It's one of the easiest ways I know to explain how the energy around us can be healing and even transformational.

I can remember the first time I received the intangible gift of Healing Touch, an energy-based therapy that restores balance and facilitates healing. I would never be the same. It was back in the 1990s, when I was still working in the cardiac catheterization lab, placing stents in diseased arteries. I had contracted disseminated herpes from a patient, and the virus had quickly spread throughout my system. It really took me down. My resiliency was very low; I had been working a grueling on-call schedule and hadn't yet discovered yoga or meditation or the healing powers of integrative medicine.

I began to miss work, which is very unusual for a physician, especially an interventional cardiologist. Around the sixth day, one of my partners called and asked if I needed to be hospitalized. I told him that I had sores all over my mouth, my glands were swollen, and my neck looked double its usual size. He immediately suggested I be admitted into the hospital for IV medication.

Then I received a second phone call, this time from my nurse, Rauni King, who was running the Ornish Program for Reversing Heart Disease. She offered to give me a Healing Touch treatment. I knew she performed this biofield technique on ICU patients, but I never thought it would help me.

As two hours of treatment went by; I barely remember Rauni even touching my body. I went into a profound state of relaxation, as if I were floating on a calm sea. I do not remember what transpired, but one thing is certain: when Rauni finished the treatment, my energy, vitality, and sense of well-being was significantly improved. I was able to get up and get dressed. The next day I went to work almost as if I had never felt bad in the first place.

I immediately wanted to learn more about Healing Touch and began to explore ways to make this treatment available to my patients. Yet that was just the beginning of my journey. Over the next seven years, I continued to have treatments myself and became a Healing Touch practitioner. Rauni began to provide Healing Touch to our patients going for cardiac catheterization and surgical procedures. Our data consistently showed reductions in pain and anxiety.

In 2010, when we were contacted by a commander at Camp Pendleton, a U.S. Marine Corps base in Southern California, asking if we had any Integrative Medicine approaches that would help active marines suffering from PTSD, we recommended Healing Touch and guided imagery. In 2012, we published our results in *Military Medicine*. We demonstrated a statistically significant reduction in PTSD and depression symptoms in marines treated with Healing Touch and guided imagery. Today, military bases around the country now use these approaches.

80. Get in Touch With Your Biofield.

Our knowledge of the healing power of energy dates back to Hippocrates, the Greek physician and father of modern medicine.

Hippocrates noted that a "force flowed from people's hands." Greek philosopher Pythagoras referred to the biofield (energy fields that surround the body) as "vital energy perceived as a luminous body that could produce cures." According to many global healing traditions, such as Ayurveda and Traditional Chinese Medicine, the biofield is in and around the physical body.

I believe that Pythagoras and Hippocrates were right, and many others agree. Numerous cultures have their own names for this vital force. The Chinese call it *chi*. Indian Ayurvedic medicine calls it *prana*. It is referred to as *ki* in Japan and *mana* in Hawaii and Polynesia.

Biofield therapies are part of the field of energy medicine, and they remain a subject of much debate in Western medicine. Conventional medical schools don't teach the anatomy of the biofield, yet nearly every global healing tradition uses biofield therapies for healing in some form: acupuncture, Tai Chi, Qigong, homeopathy, Healing Touch, and others. Ample evidence shows that biofield therapies have a positive impact on health.

Biofield practitioners believe that the energy system has three key components: the chakras, meridians, and aura. There are seven major chakras, or energy centers, in the body, positioned from the base of the spine to the crown. (In Sanskrit, *chakra* means spinning wheel or vortex.) Meridians are energy tracts that run along the body from head to toe, and these are often the focus of such energy treatments as acupuncture and acupressure. The aura is the energy field that surrounds the entire body. In the Christian tradition, the biofield appears as a halo.

Practitioners of energy medicine work within different regions of the biofield. For example, acupuncturists place needles in the energy tracts or meridians, while Healing Touch practitioners work on the aura and chakra systems.

Biofield treatments remain outside of Western medicine's toolbox. Why can't physicians agree on whether energy medicine is effective? One of the key reasons is that we don't have technology that reproducibly measures the biofield or allows us to see it in a tangible way. But this does not mean it does not exist!

Experience Your Energy Field

One of the best ways to understand the idea of biofield therapies is to learn to feel your own energy field. Tap into it with this
simple, five-minute exercise:

- **Sit in a comfortable chair** with your feet flat on
  the ground.

- **Take a few slow, deep breaths,** breathing five
  seconds in and five seconds out.

- **Close your eyes and imagine** roots growing from the
  soles of your feet and anchoring into the earth's core.
  Imagine these roots anchoring at the earth's center.
  Now, slowly pull up the energy from the earth into
  the soles of your feet. Allow the energy to slowly rise
  past your ankles and your knees and into your hips.
  Slowly pull the energy up and let it fill your lower
  extremities. Allow the energy to come up into your
  spine, starting at the base. Now, move the energy
  upward to below the navel, into your solar plexus,
  and then into your heart center. Imagine your heart
  center filled with a beautiful, radiant light. Allow
  this light to expand at your heart's center, then move
  down your arms and into the palms of your hands.
  Remember to continue to breathe as you conduct
  this exercise.

- **Now, gently cup your hands and bring them
  toward each other; do not let them touch.** When
  your hands are about eight inches apart, gently
  expand and contract the space between them. Slowly
  you will begin to feel the electromagnetic field. It
  may feel dense, thick, or like a magnet.

Don't be discouraged if you don't feel your biofield right away.
If you keep trying this exercise, you will soon experience your
own energy system.

81. Every Day, Open Each of Your Chakras.

There are seven major chakras, or energy centers, in the body. Each chakra interfaces with the physical body and can influence organs and endocrine glands such as the adrenals or thyroid. Thus, each chakra can affect your physical, emotional, mental, and spiritual well-being. When the flow of energy in one or more of the chakras becomes blocked, illness related to that energy center may result. Many energy medicine techniques focus on opening or unblocking chakras.

These are the seven major chakras:

- **The root chakra,** located at the base of the spine, is associated with basic survival needs and feeling grounded, as well as our sense of belonging. Physically, the root chakra is connected to our legs, feet, and hips. The adrenal gland is associated with this chakra.

- **The sacral chakra,** located about an inch below the navel in the reproductive area, is associated with creativity and birth. Second chakra illnesses are usually related to the reproductive system. Since this is our emotional center, illnesses in this region are typically related to our relationships.

- **The solar plexus chakra,** located in our upper abdomen and stomach, is associated with our will, self-esteem, and sense of personal accomplishment. The pancreas, stomach, and spleen are third chakra organs. Issues of self-worth and self-esteem will result in third chakra illnesses. How many times have you said, "That comment hit me in the gut"?

- **The heart chakra,** located in the chest, is associated with love, compassion, and forgiveness. When people have illnesses related to the heart chakra, they are usually related to love and loss. We use heart-related expressions all the time: "He died of a broken heart" or "My heart is broken into a million pieces." Heart disease and breast cancer are classic fourth chakra illnesses. The lungs surround this chakra, and lung issues are frequently related to grief.

- **The throat chakra,** located right at the thyroid gland, is associated with self-expression and speaking one's truth. Fifth chakra illness is usually related to the thyroid or parathyroid glands.

- **The third eye chakra,** located in the center of the forehead, is associated with information, intuition, and wisdom. The pituitary gland, eyes, and sinuses are associated with the sixth chakra. Health challenges related to the sixth chakra usually manifest in the ears, nose, eyes, and sinus.

- **The crown chakra,** located at the top of the head, is associated with higher consciousness and spiritual enlightenment. It is our connection to our higher self. The gland associated with this chakra is the pineal gland. Physical challenges with this chakra may include depression, alienation, or a feeling of disconnection and confusion.

When I first learned about the chakras, I was eager to apply my new knowledge in treating my patients. Naturally, though, I was skeptical at first. I wanted to determine if there truly was an association between the chakras and health. So I began to ask my patients a lot of questions.

If someone has challenges with her thyroid, I always ask: "Is there something you are not saying? Are you speaking your truth?" If reproductive health challenges occur, I always ask about relationships, sex, intimacy, and children.

You can open and balance your chakras to enhance your health. Each morning before getting out of bed, open your seven major chakras. You will find that doing this practice daily helps you feel more balanced physically, mentally, emotionally, and spiritually. Healing Touch instructors believe that this simple technique also helps to prevent illness.

To begin, place one hand over your genital region and the second below your navel, holding your hands one inch above your body. These are your first and second chakras. As you place your hands over each chakra, imagine love pouring out of your hands and into the chakra. After two to three minutes, remove the lower hand from the genital area and place it over the third chakra, located in the gut region right below the breastbone. Next, remove the hand below your navel and place it over your heart. Each time you change a hand position, hold the new position for a few minutes. You will always have both hands over your body. Next, move the lower hand over your throat region. Then move your heart chakra hand to over your third eye, which is situated in the center of your forehead. The last position is the crown chakra at the top of your head. At the end of the sequence, one hand is on the crown and one is over the third eye. Simply let your hands walk up your chakras. Remember, hold each position for two or three minutes. This exercise will help you feel more balanced and grounded for the day.

82. Give Acupuncture a Try.

I always have a full-time acupuncturist in my cardiology practice. In fact, just about every integrative medicine center in the country has an acupuncturist. Even the Department of Defense utilizes acupuncture right on the battlefield. Why would a cardiologist want an office full of acupuncturists?

For me, it started with a frozen shoulder. After a simple injury, I was barely able to lift my right arm above my head. An orthopedic surgeon suggested a steroid injection, which I reluctantly agreed to. Unfortunately, the steroids didn't work. A friend suggested I see a Traditional Chinese Medicine physician on my next trip to New York City. Much to my surprise, Dr. Co's office was located in the back room of a hair salon on Madison Avenue. After a quick exam, he said he would perform acupressure on my back and shoulder; I would need to return the next day for acupuncture. I agreed. Within 24 hours, my frozen shoulder was cured. And I have not looked back since. If acupuncture, like Healing Touch, could heal me, then I wanted acupuncture available for my patients.

Pain is a chief complaint of many of my patients. Of course, I want to relieve their pain in the most harmless way possible. Many over-the-counter medicines, like ibuprofen, cause ulcers, kidney disease, and high blood pressure when used on a long-term basis. When I established the Scripps Center for Integrative Medicine, I wanted to offer our patients a different option. I chose acupuncture.

For more than 2,500 years, acupuncture has been a key component of Traditional Chinese Medicine. It is based on important energy concepts, most notably those of yin and yang. The yin and yang pairing explores the important coexistence and necessary balance of opposites—light and dark, male and female—not only in the universe, but within each individual.

Traditional Chinese Medicine believes that *chi*, or energy, circulates through the energy meridians that cover the body. If chi is blocked or deficient along a meridian, it can cause illness. Acupuncture techniques attempt to eliminate the illness by manipulating acupuncture points along the meridians to restore the flow of chi.

In 1998, the National Institutes of Health issued a statement endorsing the use of acupuncture for a number of conditions, including elbow tendonitis, plantar fasciitis, muscle spasm, nausea, high blood pressure, infertility, asthma, and addiction. I have recommended acupuncture to my patients for all these conditions and more.

Today, functional Magnetic Resonance Imaging (fMRI) and positron emission imaging (PET) can help us to understand how acupuncture works. With these technologies, we can visualize the brain in real time as acupuncture needles are placed. The results are compelling. Researchers are now starting to map the biofield, determining which areas of the brain are affected by acupuncture point stimulation. For example, for years, acupuncturists treated dry mouth (xerostomia) by placing acupuncture needles in certain meridians on the body. They decided to use fMRI to determine if the traditional needle insertion causes brain regions to be activated. What they found was that while sham or fake acupuncture had no effect on brain function, true acupuncture caused the insula region of the brain to light up on fMRI. The brain signaling changes were associated with saliva production.

Acupuncture can benefit many conditions. Osteoarthritis of the knee, muscle spasm, asthma, nausea, tension headache, and migraine are a few examples. Acupuncture can also be used to relieve pain and promote a deep state of relaxation. To learn more, speak with a health-care practitioner who understands the benefits of acupuncture. Work with a Traditional Chinese Medicine physician or a licensed acupuncturist who has extensive training. Many websites can help you find an acupuncturist in your area, including those of the American Association of Acupuncture and Oriental Medicine (www.aaaomonline.org) and the American Academy of Medical Acupuncture (www.medicalacupuncture. org). Find a practitioner certified by the National Certification Commission for Acupuncture and Oriental Medicine (NCCAOM) as a Diplomate of Oriental Medicine (Dipl.O.M.) or Diplomate of Acupuncture (Dipl.Ac.).

83. Explore the Healing Energy of Touch.

I have been using Healing Touch in my practice since 1996. Healing Touch practitioners use touch to positively influence the biofield that surrounds the body by clearing disruptions in the human energy system. They believe that such disruptions can lead to illness and must be cleared for healing to take place. The practice was developed in the 1980s by a nurse named Janet Mentgen. Since then, it has been extensively endorsed by the American Holistic Nurses Association and taught all over the world.

In my own practice, Rauni King and I evaluated Healing Touch in 200 patients before and after bypass surgery. We found that Healing Touch helped to relieve their fear, decrease their pain, and decrease their anxiety.

Earlier, I mentioned a 2010 study that we conducted with active marines who had been diagnosed with PTSD. The marines were randomly placed in either a control group or a group that received Healing Touch and guided imagery. Those assigned to Healing Touch and guided imagery had a statistically significant reduction in their PTSD symptoms and a reduction in depression. The most difficult part of this study was that all the marines wanted treatment; none wanted to be in the control group.

As I noted, the military is now making Healing Touch available to soldiers returning from war. At the Veterans Administration hospital in West Los Angeles, Rauni has taught Healing Touch to more than 200 nurses and health-care providers.

Anyone can learn Healing Touch. Visit www.HTI.org to find a class near your location. Even the Level 1 class will provide you with many techniques for healing both yourself and others. I strongly encourage parents to learn Healing Touch; it provides wonderful techniques for when children are injured or sick.

84. Feel the Energy Flow Through Your Body with Tai Chi.

Nearly every morning, if you walk along the cliffs overlooking the ocean in La Jolla, California, you'll likely see a woman in her 60s standing alone, moving her entire body gently and fluidly, as if she can hear some music the rest of us are not privy to. It almost looks like she is doing a slow-motion dance. Her expression is calm, and she seems to be completely and contentedly focused on her movements.

This carefully choreographed routine, called Tai Chi, is coordinated with the breath to release both physical and emotional stress. According to Traditional Chinese Medicine, Tai Chi and Qigong promote the flow of energy through the body. The exercises incorporate deep relaxation techniques, breathing exercises, self-massage, and even stimulation of acupuncture points without needles. I remember that during my first trip to China in 2001, it was not unusual to see hundreds of people in the park each morning performing Tai Chi exercises. People who practice Tai Chi regularly report feeling stronger, relaxed, and revitalized.

Studies have found that Tai Chi improves balance, muscle strength, endurance, and flexibility. It decreases blood pressure and improves heart rate variability, both of which are risk factors for heart disease and stroke. A study conducted in 2005 randomly assigned 30 patients with congestive heart failure to a group that practiced Tai Chi versus conventional care. Individuals in the Tai Chi group demonstrated marked improvement in their quality of life, strength, and flexibility.

Many of my patients enjoy this form of exercise, which is a combination of physical activity and mind-body medicine. There are many resources available to help you learn Tai Chi, including live classes, online videos, DVDs, and books. Search online for classes in your area. There are five main Tai Chi forms. I recommend short-form styles to start, especially for people who are older and new to martial arts. For individuals with knee and lower back challenges, forms with higher rather than lower stances are preferred. Speak to the instructor before taking a class, and let them know if you have any physical limitations.

85. Try Homeopathic Remedies.

When you were growing up, your mother or father may have kept a small bottle of a liquid called ipecac in the first-aid kit. This terrible-tasting liquid was used to induce vomiting when someone swallowed something poisonous. (Due to its potentially dangerous side effets, ipecac syrup is no longer recommended for home use.) However, in homeopathic medicine, ipecac serves the opposite purpose. An extremely diluted solution of ipecac is used to treat nausea rather than induce it.

Hippocrates said, "Through the like disease is produced, and through the like disease is cured." *Homos* in Greek means "similar," and *pathos* means "suffering." Homeopathy is a natural biofield science based on this "like cures like" theory—according to it, an energized medicine that mimics a symptom promotes healing and relieves the symptom. Homeopathy uses very small and often highly diluted doses of plants, minerals, and animal materials to stimulate the immune system and facilitate healing.

Skeptics find it hard to believe that such tiny doses can have any significant effect on healing, but research shows otherwise. In 1991, the *British Medical Journal* published a meta-analysis of 107 controlled trials using homeopathy; the researchers concluded that 81 were effective, 24 were ineffective, and two were inconclusive. The researchers concluded that these positive results warrant further investigation and consideration of homeopathy for certain conditions.

The rest of the world seems to agree. India has 125 homeopathic medical schools. Homeopathy is taught in German medical schools and used by German physicians. In England, 42 percent of general practitioners refer patients to homeopaths. While I don't consider myself a homeopath, I use many of the basic remedies in my practice. I refer my more advanced patients to a specialist in homeopathic medicine.

Give homeopathy a try. There are many wonderful natural treatments that are safe to use at home, even for children. Arnica montana, for example, helps to soothe muscle aches, treat bruises, and reduce inflammation. In fact, it is prescribed by most cosmetic surgeons and considered to be as effective as nonsteroidal anti-inflammatory agents like ibuprofen. (See Appendix F for a toolbox of basic homeopathic remedies.)

• ● •

CHAPTER 12

One World: Preserve Your Health, Protect the Planet

In 2000, more than 1,300 scientists, authors, and reviewers worldwide contributed their knowledge, time, and insight to the Millennium Ecosystem Assessment. This project aimed to provide a scientific appraisal of the world's ecosystems and the resources they provide, such as food, clean water, and natural resources, and then to establish a scientific basis for action to conserve and sustain them for all forms of life.

The findings were deeply disturbing. According to the Millennium Assessment Report, 25 percent of mammals and 30 percent of amphibians are threatened with extinction. Two-thirds of major marine fisheries are fully exploited or worse. And one billion people lack access to fresh, clean water. To quote the Millennium Assessment: "At the heart of this assessment is a stark warning: Human activity is putting such strain on the natural functions of Earth that the ability of the planet's ecosystems to sustain future generations can no longer be taken for granted."

Ecology is the study of all interconnected systems on the planet. We must recognize that we are part of the web of life; what happens to one part of the web happens to all. Climate change, agricultural industrialization, and the extensive use of synthetic chemicals and plastics impact the health of our planet, which then impacts the health of humanity. Human health is intimately connected to the health of the planet; what is personal is truly universal.

86. Take Control of Your Toxin Exposure.

In 1970, the United States Environmental Protection Agency (EPA) was formed to regulate the production, use, and disposal of chemicals in the United States. This was followed by the Toxic Substances Control Act (TSCA) of 1976, which states: "It is the policy of the United States that adequate data should be developed with respect to the effect of chemical substances and mixtures on health and the environment."

Sounds great, right? Unfortunately, the TSCA continues: "The development of such data should be the responsibility of those who manufacture and those who process such chemical substances and mixtures." So instead of an outside, objective agency evaluating and regulating the safety of toxins, the job was given to those who make money by manufacturing them. The TSCA in 1976 grandfathered in approximately 62,000 chemicals, despite the lack of safety data to support this policy.

This might help explain why, in the past four decades, only five classes of synthetic chemicals have been banned in the United States due to concerns about human and environmental health. One of these chemicals was the organochloride pesticide DDT. The United States banned DDT in 1972 after the widely used pesticide was found to be accumulating in animal tissues and threatening endangered species, including the bald eagle and peregrine falcon.

But what about the other toxins we don't even know about? There are all kinds of chemicals in mass production, and very little is known about the toxicity of many of them. The 1998 EPA Chemical Hazard Data Availability Study says: "EPA's analysis found that no basic toxicity information, i.e., neither human health nor environmental toxicity, is publicly available for 43 percent of the high volume chemicals manufactured in the U.S. and that a full set of basic toxicity information is available for only 7 percent of these chemicals."

More current research links exposure to harmful chemicals to a number of serious health concerns. The EPA's 2008 *Report on the Environment* states: "Exposure to environmental contaminants has been linked to many human diseases and conditions, including cancer, cardiovascular disease, respiratory disease, some infectious diseases and low birth weight."

The good news is that we are at a turning point. It is now recognized that toxins are associated with many diseases, including cancer, birth defects, and infertility. Campaigns for kid-safe chemicals have created a large national consensus for change. The current bills before Congress call for a demonstration of safety for all chemicals that were grandfathered in by 1976 law. The bills state that new chemicals must be safe for children and all vulnerable groups. In addition, information about chemicals must be made public.

The nonprofit, nonpartisan Environmental Working Group (EWG) is raising awareness about this issue and placing education and tools in our hands to help us make clear, informed decisions. Visit their site at www.ewg.org for a wealth of great information to help you and your loved ones avoid common household toxins and choose toxin-free cosmetics, produce, seafood, and much more.

Support Your Liver to Minimize Damage from Toxins

You can help minimize the damage from environmental toxins by supporting your liver, the major organ involved in detoxification. The following are my favorite fruits and vegetables that help turn on liver enzymes that enhance this process:

- Artichokes
- Brussels sprouts
- Cabbage
- Basil
- Oregano
- Parsley
- Pinto and red beans
- Oranges
- Tomatoes
- Arugula
- Kale
- Bok choy
- Mustard greens

I also recommend the following supplements for liver support:

- Milk thistle, 300 milligrams per day
- N-acetylcysteine (NAC), 600 milligrams per day
- Omega-3 (EPA/DHA) fish oil, 1,000 milligrams per day

87. Know How Your Food Was Raised.

Wouldn't it be great if cattle could roam freely over wide open plains, spending all day in the fresh air, grazing on green grass? Sadly, cattle are usually kept on feedlots in confined quarters, often without enough room to simply turn around. They are fattened up with hormones until they are ready for market. Chickens are raised in similar conditions.

Because these animals are kept in such cramped and oppressive housing, farmers routinely give them antibiotics to prevent infection. Notice that I used the word "prevent" and not "treat." Animals routinely get antibiotics and hormones they do not even need. Rather than offer conditions that might keep the animals healthy—such as fresh air, sunlight, and room to roam freely ("free-range")—they are given powerful drugs in their food and water. Imagine if we gave all our school children antibiotics every day so that they wouldn't get sick from being in the classroom together!

The agricultural industry uses more than 70 percent of the antibiotics produced in the United States—and there is a strong link between antibiotics used in agriculture and the growing prevalence of antibiotic-resistant bacteria. A report from 2000 traced an outbreak of antibiotic-resistant salmonella in the United Kingdom to a dairy farm where a particular antibiotic had been used in the previous month. In 1987, a similar study reportedly traced tetracycline-resistant salmonella back to cattle feed. In both cases, antibiotics added to the animals' food and water resulted in antibiotic-resistant infection in humans.

The WHO 2016 fact sheet warns "antibiotic resistance is rising to dangerously high levels in all parts of the world. New resistance mechanisms are emerging and spreading globally, threatening our ability to treat common infectious diseases." The American Society for Microbiology, the American Public Health Association, and the American Medical Association have all called for substantial restrictions on antibiotic use in animals, including an end to all preventive use of antibiotics in livestock. In 2011, a letter signed by professional medical organizations and sent to Congress stated: "The evidence is so strong of a link between misuse of antibiotics and food, or in animal food, and human antibiotic resistance that FDA and Congress should be acting much more boldly and urgently to protect those vital drugs for human illness."

Hormones are creating another problem. Hormones can make animals grow faster and produce more milk. In 1993, the FDA approved the use of recombinant bovine growth hormone (rBGH) in cows to increase milk production. Cows treated with growth hormone frequently develop an infection called mastitis, which then requires antibiotics for treatment. This hormone is banned in the European Union, Canada, and other countries.

The easiest way to avoid hormones? *Eat a vegan diet.* Remember, if you eat an animal, you will be affected by whatever that animal ate. Or, look for the Certified Humane Raised and Handled label. Certified Humane Raised and Handled food products come from facilities that meet high standards for farm animal treatment. If you are a vegetarian who consumes dairy and eggs, choose organic.

I suggest that everyone buy organic fruits and vegetables as well, especially if they are on the Dirty Dozen list I discussed in Chapter 3.

How You Can Help Control the Spread of Antibiotic Resistance

1. Only use antibiotics when prescribed by a certified health professional. Never demand antibiotics if your health practitioner says they are not necessary.

2. Always follow your health practitioner's advice when antibiotics are prescribed. Never share leftover antibiotics or randomly take them without guidance

3. Speak with an integrative health practitioner; there is a good chance they will have recommendations to boost your immune system and fight infections.

4. Prevent infections: wash your hands, prepare food hygienically, avoid close contact with sick people, and practice safe sex.

88. Filter Your Water.

Tap or bottled? Seems like an innocuous enough question, one that we are often asked when we dine out. Yet, increasingly, we aren't quite sure how to answer it. The truth is, the best option is always filtered water, which may or may not come from a tap but should never come from a plastic bottle.

Not only is plastic bad for the environment, but bottled water is not necessarily less contaminated. It may not even be filtered! Knowing your water source is critical to knowing potential contaminants. Say no to bottled water whenever possible.

It is best to filter your own water and carry it in stainless steel containers. Hard plastic bottles (#7 plastic) can leach a harmful chemical called bisphenol-A (BPA) right into your water. Carry BPA-free or stainless steel bottles. Never reuse plastic water bottles.

In North America, water toxins can vary across national borders and from state to state. When the Environmental Working Group studied the drinking water in 35 U.S. cities in 2010, they analyzed for the first time the presence of the chemical hexavalent chromium in the water systems. Measurable amounts of this chemical, a known carcinogen, were found in the tap water of 31 of the cities sampled; 25 of these cities had levels that exceeded the limit recommended by the EPA.

Researchers at the Environmental Working Group have identified 316 chemicals in U.S. tap water, and many of these are unregulated.

With so many potential contaminants, we should all be filtering our water. But before you invest in a simple or complex water filter system, check out what contaminants are common in your state. The EWG website hosts a state-by-state National Drinking Water Database. I was shocked to learn that my hometown of San Diego ranked 92 out of 100—close to the lowest-rated water utility in the country—and averages 20 pollutants in the water compared to the national average of 8. Other cities, like Arlington, Texas, rank near the top.

When picking a water filtering system, follow these steps:

- Do your research on the type of filter you need for your water supply. Different filters do different things. For example, carbon filters, usually found in pitchers and faucet devices, are excellent at removing lead and by-products from water treatment applications. Reverse osmosis filters are needed to remove arsenic.

- Check out the National Water Database (www. ewg.org/tap-water) for your area to learn which contaminants are of greatest concern for you.

- Purchase a filter that fits your needs. This may be a simple pitcher or faucet filter or a more complex whole-home filtration system.

- Remember to change your water filters as scheduled.

89. Reduce Your Carbon Footprint.

Greenhouse gases are gases that trap heat in the atmosphere. According to the EPA, carbon dioxide makes up 82 percent of all greenhouse gas emissions in the United States. Globally, carbon dioxide makes up 57 percent of all greenhouse gas emissions, with the majority coming from the burning of coal, natural gas, and oil for heat and electricity. The agricultural industry accounts for 14 percent—more than transportation, wastewater, and residential buildings. Trees absorb carbon dioxide; deforestation can account for 5 billion metric tons of carbon dioxide emissions.

A carbon footprint is the amount of carbon dioxide or other carbon compounds emitted into the atmosphere by the activities of an individual, company, country, and so on. It describes the impact of carbon emissions on the environment. About 80 percent of the world's energy is from carbon-based sources: coal, oil, and gas. The quickest action to combat climate change that we can take is to immediately eliminate the use of coal.

The EPA offers a carbon footprint calculator on its website (www.epa.gov). Assess your carbon footprint and implement some easy ways to reduce it. According to the EPA, the following are some of the ways you can improve yours:

- Eat less meat. The agricultural industry has one of the biggest carbon and water footprints. Start a campaign for meatless Mondays and Fridays.

- Change your lightbulbs to those that have the Energy Star label.

- Power down your electronics when you aren't using them.

- Look for the WaterSense label when purchasing items for your home such as bathroom sink faucets, showerheads, and toilets.

- Compost your vegetable waste. This reduces waste going to landfills, helping to decrease their greenhouse gas emissions.

- Insulate and seal your home.

- Don't leave the water running.

- Collect rainwater for gardening.

- Take shorter showers and don't consume gallons of water in a bath.

- Reduce, reuse, recycle. Sometimes it is better to *refuse*—like refusing to use plastic bags and bottles.

- Plant a tree. Reforestation or the planting of trees is critically important to mitigating the effect of greenhouse gases. The larger the tree, the more carbon dioxide it will absorb.

- Use drip irrigation on your property or plant a drought-tolerant landscape.

90. Shop at Your Local Co-Op.

A cooperative (co-op) is a business owned by its members, for the benefit of its members. For example, a consumer co-op may provide food, health care, housing, and financial services for its members. A credit union is an example of a co-op. The average co-op employs 90 members of the community and has a profoundly positive impact on community development and prosperity.

Food co-ops are committed to providing high-quality products that are local, organic, and natural. The goal is to enhance the well-being and health of its members, the community, and the environment. Food co-ops purchase more food from local farmers than conventional grocers do. Local farmers, in turn, buy their supplies from local sources and hire local people to repair equipment and provide other services.

It is estimated that for every $1,000 a shopper spends at their local food co-op, $1,604 in local economic activity is generated. On average, a co-op worker is more likely to have benefits and earn $1 more per hour than conventional grocery store workers. In addition, co-ops recycle 81 percent of plastic, 96 percent of cardboard, and 74 percent of food products, which is significantly more than conventional grocers do.

Visit the Cooperative Grocer website (www.ncga.coop/find -co-op) to find a co-op near you.

91. Be a Conscious Consumer.

Where and how you spend your money matters. Your money can empower programs that support human rights while improving the health of the planet. Look at the foods in your grocery cart and check for these two labels:

The **Fair Trade** label. It is granted to products that are produced by workers and farmers who are justly compensated for their work. Fair Trade USA is a nonprofit organization that helps developing countries build businesses that are sustainable and improve the community. More than 12,000 products bearing the Fair Trade label are sourced from more than 70 developing countries throughout the world, including countries in Africa, Asia, the Caribbean, and Latin America.

The **Fair Food Program** label. The Fair Food Program is a human rights program that is monitored, enforced, and designed by the workers whose rights it was created to protect. All the food purchased under the Fair Food label is grown under policies that monitor for sexual harassment, child labor, and slavery. Many farm workers live in substandard housing and work for $2 or less per day. The Fair Food Program helps ensure that workers picking fruits and vegetables on farms are paid a fair wage and are provided with humane working conditions.

Make a conscious effort to slowly increase the number of ethically produced foods you choose, even starting with one or two. When possible, choose to shop from merchants that purchase Fair Food products. These include many large corporations like Chipotle (2012), Trader Joe's (2012), and Walmart (2014). McDonald's and Subway were early adopters, participating in the Fair Food Program since 2007 and 2008. Here are a few websites to get you started:

- The Coalition of Immokalee Workers' (CIW) Fair Food Program: www.fairfoodprogram.org

- Fair Trade USA: www.fairtradeusa.org

- Ecolabel Index: www.ecolabelindex.com

The EcoLabels website provides a full listing of every label from Organic to Certified Humane and Dolphin Safe. Visit this site and familiarize yourself with the labels; this will help you to recognize these products in the store.

92. Avoid PVC: The "Poison Plastic."

PVC, or polyvinyl chloride, is by far the most environmentally damaging plastic. According to the Environmental Justice fact sheet, PVC plants in the United States pump some 500,000 pounds of vinyl chloride—a known human carcinogen—and many other toxins into the atmosphere annually. The entire PVC life cycle— from production to use to disposal—causes the release of toxic, chlorine-containing chemicals. These toxins are now building up in our food chain, air, and water.

PVC can be found almost everywhere, from packaging and children's toys to automobile parts and building materials. A majority of PVC plants are found in the poorer areas of Texas and Louisiana. In 1987, the town of Reveilletown, Louisiana, became so contaminated that all 106 residents were relocated and every building was torn down. Studies have documented links between working in PVC facilities and the increased likelihood of developing diseases such as angiosarcoma, liver and lung cancer, leukemia, and lymphoma.

The only way to avoid PVC is to look for a triangle made up of arrows on your plastic items. If the number in the center of the triangle is a 3, your plastic is PVC and should be avoided. Shop for PVC-free products and encourage local schools and building to be constructed without PVC.

93. Beware of Mercury: Choose
Fish and Seafood Carefully.

Fish is rich in omega-3s, which lowers triglyceride levels, reduces blood pressure, and fights inflammation. Sounds like a healthy option for your heart, right? Unfortunately, there's a hidden side to coronary artery disease; it's not related simply to high cholesterol. Many of my patients are aware of this and have had advanced testing for both cholesterol and inflammatory markers. However, very few have been checked for heavy metals.

When David came to see me after a cardiac arrest, he'd already had seven stents. He explained that even after 20 cholesterol checks, angiograms, and echocardiograms, he thought something had been missed. He was right. His heavy metals had never been checked. And his mercury level was off the charts.

We now know that methyl mercury is toxic to the heart as well as to the brain, kidney, liver, and nervous system. Mercury toxicity is associated with nervous system damage, sleep disturbance, headache, fatigue, and difficulty with memory and concentration. David had many of these symptoms in addition to coronary artery disease. The key to preventing further coronary disease in David was not in treating his cholesterol but in chelating his mercury!

When you eat fish, be smart about the choices you make:

- Choose fish high in omega-3 and low in mercury. Mercury bioaccumulates in larger fish, so stick with wild salmon, Atlantic mackerel, mussels, sardines, and rainbow trout. Oysters, herring, and anchovy are okay as well.

- Avoid high-mercury fish: shark, swordfish, king mackerel, tilefish, marlin, orange roughy, and bluefin tuna.

- Go to www.seafoodwatch.org or download the Seafood Watch mobile app for up-to-date information on seafood.

Is Wild Salmon Really Better Than Farm Raised?

Yes. Without question. A 2004 study published in *Science* found that farm-raised Atlantic salmon had significantly higher levels of 13 toxins when compared with wild Pacific salmon. The study also measured toxin levels in the salmon chow, which is the mixture of ground-up fish and oil fed to the farm-raised salmon. Researchers found a strong correlation between the toxicities of the chow and the salmon, and they concluded that the toxins were being passed into the salmon from their food.

Although mercury exposure can come from many sources, including dental fillings, fish is the common culprit. To address this issue as well as the issue of sustainability, the Monterey Bay Aquarium launched its Seafood Watch program in 1999. The purpose of Seafood Watch is to provide scientifically based recommendations for the best seafood to consume based on sustainability and mercury content. A Seafood Watch "green" rating or "best choice" goes to sources of fish that are "well managed and caught or farmed in ways that cause little harm to habitats or other wildlife." A "yellow" rating is given to species with "some concerns" for sustainability. "Red" ratings are for fish to avoid. For example, high grades are given for sustainability to farmed scallops, oysters, mussels, Arctic char, striped bass, catfish, and rainbow trout. But salmon and shrimp farming often damage surrounding ecosystems and receive a much lower rating.

94. Beware of BPA.

You may have heard about bisphenol A (BPA) in the news. It is an industrial chemical that has been used to make plastics and resins since the 1960s. The two main sources of BPA are the linings inside cans of food and rigid plastics made of polycarbonate, such as water and baby bottles, sippy cups, and sports bottles. The concern is that the BPA in these containers can seep into our food. The Harvard School of Public Health has reported a link between high BPA exposure and consumption of canned soup.

Even some baby toys are made of BPA—and babies put everything into their mouths.

Early research has linked BPA exposure to heart disease, diabetes, learning disabilities, and obesity. BPA is an endocrine disruptor and can behave in a similar way to estrogen and other hormones in the human body. Early child development is the time of greatest sensitivity to the negative impacts of BPA. Studies have linked prenatal exposure to later neurological challenges in children.

Canada was the first to ban BPA from baby bottles in 2008. Both the U.S. Department of Health and Human Services and the FDA have expressed some concerns about the possible health effects of BPA. In July 2012, BPA was finally banned from baby bottles and sippy cups here.

The following tips will help you avoid BPA as much as possible:

- Avoid plastic containers with the number 3 or 7 in the recycling symbol on the bottom.

- Do not microwave plastic food containers made of polycarbonate.

- Limit your use of canned foods, which frequently have BPA in the lining of the can.

- Use glass, stainless steel, or porcelain containers.

- Use stainless steel water bottles.

- Do not use aluminum bottles, because many are lined with BPA.

- Avoid bottles that contain BPS and BPF, which are substitutes for BPA. Concerns have been raised by researchers that these substitutes also have the potential to behave as endocrine disruptors.

95. Plastic Is Forever. Stop Filling Our Oceans With It.

There are two areas in the North Pacific Ocean known as the Great Pacific Garbage Patches. These areas contain trash vortexes—gyres of ocean litter. The Eastern Garbage Patch is midway between Hawaii and California, and the Western Garbage Patch is off the coast of Japan.

The term *garbage patch* is a bit of a misnomer. These patches don't merely float on the surface; instead, the debris is mixed in with the currents and is often not even visible from above. But the garbage is there, and it is growing. New patches are forming as well. According to the National Oceanic and Atmospheric Administration, the main ingredient in these patches is plastic debris.

All that plastic is killing our sea life and contaminating our oceans. Sea turtles mistake plastic bags for jellyfish, try to eat them, and end up with plastic entwined in their internal organs, leading to a slow and painful death. Dolphins and seabirds do the same. Birds, otters, and other small mammals get stuck inside plastic six-pack rings and die. Albatrosses on the Midway Atoll are dying from consuming plastic, especially bottle caps. In addition to floating in the water, ocean plastic breaks down into tiny fibers, or microplastics, and is eaten by birds and marine life. It is estimated that every square kilometer of deep ocean has four billion plastic fibers in it!

As if that's not bad enough, here are a few more ways plastic hurts the environment: It takes 17 billion barrels of oil to produce the 30 billion plastic bottles Americans use annually. In the process, 2.5 billion tons of carbon dioxide pollution are produced. It takes three times the amount of water to produce the bottle as it does to fill it. Now add to that the cost and pollution of transporting those heavy bottles.

I am thrilled that Hawaii has set the stage for the rest of the country by being the first state to ban single-use plastic bags at checkout counters. It is clear that, even with "recycling" programs, too many are ending up in the ocean. More than 1,000 cities have followed suit. Unfortunately, in some areas, single-use plastic bags have been replaced by thicker, "reusable" plastic bags that are even more damaging to the environment and are rarely used more than a few times.

Recycling is not a sustainable solution for plastic waste. Recycling plastic is costly and does not reduce the production of new plastic products. Some biodegradable plastics that can break down in landfills will not necessarily do so in water. Even biodegradable plastics do not ever fully disappear but rather break down into smaller and smaller pieces that contaminate the water and soil. Most of our plastic waste is landfilled, downcycled, or exported to other countries.

Here's what you can do to help:

- Do not buy plastic bottles, whether they contain water, soda, or any other product

- Filter your water at home. Pour it into a stainless steel bottle to take with you.

- Use reusable, washable cloth bags for shopping.

- If you have a choice between a heavily packaged product and one that does not use a lot of plastic, make the environmentally smart choice.

- Pick up and properly discard plastic waste so that it does not end up in our waterways.

- Remember: plastic is forever. Stop using plastic bottles and bags.

96. Don't Catch the "Teflon Flu." Stay Away from PFCs and Flame Retardants.

Perfluorinated chemicals (PFCs) are a family of fluorine-containing chemicals with unique properties that make materials resistant to sticking and staining. The most notable product is Teflon, marketed as a coating for nonstick pans.

Chemicals from the PFC family are associated with elevated cholesterol, thyroid dysfunction, and low-birth-weight babies. "Teflon flu" is a diagnosis given to individuals who develop flu-like symptoms after exposure to heated Teflon pans; Teflon releases chemical fumes even at moderate temperatures. These fumes have been shown to kill birds and are therefore dangerous to wildlife.

A joint research study was conducted between Duke University and the EWG to assess for the presence of chemical flame retardants in children and mothers. These flame retardants are found in car seats, baby carriers, and portable mattresses. The researchers assessed the volunteer subjects' urine for a TDCIPP metabolite. TDCIPP, a cancer-causing fire retardant, was found in the bodies of all 48 mothers and their children tested. Children ingest significantly more fire-retardant chemicals than their mothers because they spend more time on the floor playing and because they put their hands and toys in their mouths.

TDCIPP and other products such as Firemaster 550 have been used as replacements for a class of fire-retardant chemicals called polybrominated diphenyl ethers, or PBDEs. Even though the use of PBDEs has significantly slowed, furniture and other products treated with them remain in people's homes. An EWG 2005 study showed that 10 out of 10 children had flame retardants in their umbilical cord blood.

Here are a few ways to avoid these chemicals:

- Don't buy packaged foods. Many food packages contain grease-repellent coatings. Examples include French fry boxes, microwave popcorn packages, and pizza boxes.

- Avoid stain-resistance treatments. Choose furniture and carpets that aren't marketed as "stain-resistant," and do not apply stain resistance products to your new purchases.

- Read labels on personal care products. Avoid products made with Teflon or products containing ingredients with the terms *fluoro* or *perfluoro*. PFCs can be found in cosmetics, nail polish, skin moisturizers, eye makeup, and even dental floss.

- Don't cook with nonstick pans or Teflon. If you do use nonstick products, be very careful not to subject them to heat above 450°F. If the nonstick coating breaks down, throw the pan away.

- Use stainless steel and iron cookware whenever possible.

- If a product has been treated with flame-resistant material, it is best to avoid its use in your home.

- Join the EWG call for a national furniture flammability standard. Go to the EWG website (www.ewg.org) and sign this simple petition.

• ● •

CHAPTER 13

It's Your Life.
Make It Matter.

I love the story about the fisherman and the businessman. The fisherman lives in a small, quiet village where he spends countless hours on the water in his small boat. He wakes with the sunrise and sleeps when the sun goes down. His life is simple and he is at peace. One day, he is approached by a businessman offering to expand his business. He tells the fisherman he will be rich enough to sit back, relax, and leisurely fish for the rest of his life. The wise fisherman says that this is exactly what he is already doing and asks the businessman, "Why would I change a thing?"

Paul Pearsall, Ph.D., was a dear friend and author of a number of inspiring books, including *The Heart's Code*. In one of his books, he asks, "Are you thriving or just surviving?" This simple yet provocative question made me stop, think, and reevaluate the way I was living my own life.

There was a time that I was spending a majority of my waking hours working to support a lifestyle I rarely got to enjoy. Think of all the people you know who rush around in a constant state of busyness without connecting to the people and things that truly matter to them. Are you one of them?

97. Escape Your Golden Cage.

I grew up in a modest home, with three generations under one roof. We shared small bedrooms and smaller bathrooms. We had one television and one car. Clothing was passed down from one sibling to another. Most of the time, we felt like we had enough.

Today, many Americans have bigger houses, bigger bathrooms, and several really big TVs. Many homes have two big cars, and thanks to leasing, some people get new ones every few years. Every day I see people trapped in what I affectionately call "the golden cage." It's a metaphor for the life we create, usually unknowingly, when we become bound to material items, unhealthy definitions of success, and societal pressure to behave in a way that may not be the essence of our true selves.

The golden cage is a state of bondage in which we are held to the material world and the world of illusion. We work harder and longer to support a lifestyle that we frequently don't have the time to enjoy. We spend less time with our loved ones. We forget about our purpose in life and find ourselves surviving rather than thriving. Trapped by the need to maintain this lifestyle, we eventually become depleted and sometimes ill: emotionally, physically, mentally, and spiritually.

In 2009, a colleague asked me to consult on a successful oncologist named Dr. May. By the time Dr. May came to my office, she was going through a stressful divorce, was raising two teenagers, and was the sole physician in her practice. She was having problems with her memory and high blood pressure. In addition, she was angry, irritated, hyperactive, and alienating the people around her.

I quickly recognized that Dr. May was spiraling toward burnout. I knew she needed to put the brakes on immediately, so I suggested a three-month medical leave of absence. She instantly objected: "No, I can't stop working. I am the sole breadwinner for my family, I have to pay the bills in my office, I have five employees, and my children are in private school."

Dr. May is a perfect example of someone trapped in the golden cage. Her lifestyle had already resulted in divorce and was now causing even more emotional, mental, and physical challenges. With her life spiraling out of control, she felt powerless. What she had to learn is that only she holds the key to unlock the cage and transform her life.

Life Outside the Golden Cage

Visualize what it is like to wake up feeling refreshed. You have a roof over your head, food on the table, and your health. Your day begins with 20 minutes of meditation followed by a healthy breakfast. You walk to a job that brings you joy because you are doing what you love to do. After working for a few hours, you take a walk and then have lunch. You work a few more hours, and by 5 P.M., you are exercising—perhaps you take a dance class. You follow this with another 20 minutes of meditation or prayer, feeling grateful for all you have. You conclude the day with a light dinner, ideally with family or friends.

Sound impossible? Says who?

98. Go After Your Life's Desires.

I can remember being in southern India, helping a group of health-care providers build a hospital, when I first heard a discussion on the human life cycle. It was defined in 40-year phases—birth to 40, 40 to 80, and 80 to 120—with each phase seen as an opportunity to achieve specific goals. (Yes, the human life-span is considered to be 120 years.)

The first 40 years of our life are typically devoted to education, creating our careers or professions, and raising a family. Our focus is on providing for the needs of loved ones and setting a stable foundation for the future. We have our home, children, jobs, friends, and community. Life is filled with activity, running from one event to the next.

Usually, we are too busy to think about the future, because we are trying to get through our day. But what happens when the children go away to school and there is less running and racing? Many people in this next phase of life feel disconnected. Their children are at college, and they are considering retiring from their employment of many years. They begin to wonder, *What is my purpose in life?*

This is a perfect time to ask, "How do I want to spend my next 40 years?" It is a time to reflect on where we have been, but also to look at our motivations and desires for where we go next.

This shift occurred for me at the age of 50. I had devoted my life to working in hospitals, being employed by a big corporation, and playing "the game" according to their rules. But when I turned 50, something changed. It was as if my soul said, "You are done with this phase of your life." I could no longer imagine myself in countless meetings where I felt like I was wasting time. That life was not serving me anymore. The 20-minute patient appointments, cutbacks on time allotted for teaching and education, and a constant emphasis on money were no longer filling my cup. I realized I was no longer philosophically aligned with the hospital system that I worked for. I also disagreed with a lot of what I observed, such as the constant adding on of medications with no real regard for lifestyle medicine, prevention, and health creation. My colleagues were excellent, but the system and what it valued were broken—badly broken.

Midlife is a great time to plan your next phase of life. And so I did. I wanted my own practice, led by my vision of healing people and changing lives through science and compassion. I wanted to spend time with my patients and have time to teach not only them but also my colleagues who, in many ways, are also suffering under the current health-care system. So I prayed for guidance and waited for the response.

And the response came in the form of a beautiful building to practice in and an impassioned stream of health seekers looking for care that embraced and extended beyond Western medicine.

In India, I learned that the years between ages 60 and 70 are considered the prime of life. To me, this is a beautiful time—where not only do you have the lessons you've learned over the past six decades, but you have the wisdom you've gained from them to truly be of service. It is also time to start thinking about the years ahead, asking the same questions again: "What are my motivations and desires? What have I missed doing because I was too busy?" It is a great time to start thinking about your legacy and contributions to the world. A time to volunteer, give scholarships to young students, serve meals to the underserved, and do whatever it is that makes your heart sing.

Get really clear about your desires. "Where am I in my life? What are my plans for the next 40 years? What are my motivations and desires?" Write them down. No matter what your age, make plans and set goals. Stay fit and flexible, and keep learning. Aging is just a state of consciousness. Know that you have a joyous life ahead.

99. Measure Success in Kindness, Service, and Caring.

We live in a world where success is often defined by money and position. We ask new acquaintances what they do for a living and draw conclusions based on their answer. What if we instead defined success as raising a child who is kind to others? What if we considered the richest people to be those with the most internal peace?

In India, where I have done service work for more than a decade, the poorest people are often doing the physically hardest jobs. In 120-degree weather, women carry heavy bricks on their heads to build a new structure while their "bosses" sit in the shade, dressed in white linen and sipping cold soda. Yet on Fridays, everyone converges on the temple for prayer, or *puja*. Does it make me more of a Christian or Hindu if I attend service, yet forget about the poor? Is the money I put in the plate enough to wipe my conscience clean?

Here are two things we can all do to find deeper meaning in our lives:

- **Redefine success.** Think about how your actions affect others and how you could be more successful in terms of kindness and service to others and the world. People always remember how you made them feel. Can you imagine defining success by kindness, compassion, patience, and giving?

- **Reevaluate the way you spend money.** How much do you really need? Can you give more?

Once you have come up with your answers to these topics, you can restructure your life to decrease stress and promote wellness and inner peace.

The funny thing about the conscious mind is that it is never satisfied. And if we are never satisfied, we can never find happiness. We always seem to want more. We purchase a new car, and we want another one two years later. We buy a state-of-the-art cell phone and want an upgrade six months later—just to get features we rarely use. Stop and think. What really matters? What do you really need? It may not be a thing or material object, but the feeling of satisfaction knowing you have helped others.

Here is how to cultivate that feeling now:

— **Stop buying so many things you don't need.** Do you really need 30 pairs of shoes? Does anyone? Sure, a new pair of shoes can make you feel happy, yet the feeling is transient. Many teenagers reflect perfect examples of this cycle. They want and want and want something until they get it. A few hours later, they want something else.

— **Imagine that what you have is enough.** You have a home to live in, food on your table, and clothes in your closet. Yet for some reason, you feel poor. What would happen if you changed your thinking? Wouldn't you feel rich if you gave something to someone who has less? Wouldn't that be enough to lead to happiness and joy? In essence, we need to count our blessings and focus on the good in our life. The more we share with others, the richer we feel.

— **Start giving more to others now.** According to the United Nations, 80 percent of the world's people barely have any wealth. They have no means to send their children to school, get health care, or have food on the table—if they have a table at all. The world's total wealth is estimated at $223 trillion. The vast majority of people have little to nothing, while the richest 1 percent has accumulated 43 percent of the world's wealth.

What about the United States? Just 1 percent of America has 40 percent of its wealth. The poorest Americans are down to pocket change, and the middle class is not much better off. There are so many ways you can serve those with less. The need is great. The opportunity is immense. If you want to feel rich, give more.

— **Strut your "stuff" by sharing it.** Look at your clothing. Peek into your closets. Is your garage packed with "stuff" you save, though you're not sure why? Is there something you can give up to someone who may need it?

You don't need to give up your lifestyle. For the price of one dinner out, you can buy two new pairs of shoes for a needy family. Instead of buying a five-dollar cup of fancy coffee, drop the money into a charitable collection box at the grocery store. You will never know how rich you can feel until you give to others—or how much good it can do for your own personal well-being.

100. Do Something That Makes Your Heart Sing.

During one of my trips to India, a young woman with metastatic breast cancer arrived to the ashram with her oncologist. He was a dear friend of mine who frequently brought his patients to India to enhance their spiritual growth. On this particular trip, this woman's spiritual teacher, Sri Narayani Amma, had asked her what the difference was between happiness and joy. When she struggled to find the answer, he told her that she would know the answer the following day.

Not knowing what to expect, the woman was surprised when the next morning, she was asked to hand out saris to the local women. As far as the eye could see, women were lined up to receive a new sari. This was a rare gift for the local women, who were too impoverished to purchase new clothing for themselves. Women came from 58 surrounding villages; many had walked miles in bare feet. As the woman handed out the saris, she was overwhelmed with joy at the happiness she was bringing to these women. As her eyes met the eyes of the women she served, she realized on a spiritual level how connected we all are, and she was able to receive their gratitude for this gift. She was an affluent woman with all that money could buy, but she realized at that moment that the happiness she received from material acquisition was nothing next to the joy that she received when she was able to bring happiness to those in need. This act of kindness made her heart sing.

Joy is with us forever; it is permanent. We never forget joy; it becomes a part of us forever. Happiness is transient and limited to the acquisition of material things that can go away in a moment. A new car or new shoes may make us happy, but frequently that happiness is short-lived. When this woman returned to New York City, she had an amazing surprise. Her cancer specialists told her that she had had a spontaneous remission. We use that term in medicine when we don't know how a cancer or other illness disappears without "proper" treatment. Some of us would call this a healing.

What gifts do you bring to this world? What makes your heart sing? When was the last time you felt joy? Your gift to the world need not be monetary. Maybe it is your time or your energy. Have you thought about volunteering? People who volunteer often experience what is known in medicine as "the helper's high." They have less depression and anxiety as well as fewer aches and pains. It feels good to do good. Do you have a skill set to volunteer in a hospital, a nursing home, or the local animal shelter? Do children need you after school to teach them to read or write? Are there refugees in your area that need assistance in integrating into our society? Do something that brings you joy and makes your heart sing, no matter how small.

As Narayani Amma said, "Whatever your worries are, whatever your sufferings are, just do good deeds. It will change your life. Dharma, good deeds and generosity, cannot be measured by quantity or by numbers. It is measured by how readily and how willingly we give to other people."

101. Make the Present Moment the Only Moment.

Hardly a day goes by where we don't find ourselves dwelling on the past or worrying about the future. We remember negative past events in painful detail and allow these memories to cloud our vision of what can be.

Our minds jump from thought to thought, from past to present to future. Remember, when we keep our thoughts to the now, the present, we are more in control of our mind.

I have a ritual that I use to let go of worries and fear. Each New Year's Eve, I write down all the things that I want to let go of in my life. I make a list and ask for forgiveness for myself and others. Then I write down my fears and worries. I burn the list in my fireplace, and I release my fears, worries, and concerns with love and light. I invite you to do the same:

- Sit quietly and make a list of your past hurts, fears, and worries.

- Set your intention on releasing these challenges and freeing yourself emotionally.

- Burn the paper and repeat, "I release past hurts, fears, and worries with love." As you burn the paper, set the intention that these emotions will be neutralized. Let them go with light and love. They may be part of your life, but they don't define who you truly are.

I love the Buddhist teaching, "Present moment, only moment." Use this mantra to keep your mind from going over past hurts and disappointments.

102. Release Your Worries: Affirm the Present Moment.

Worrying about the future is like watching a cat sitting on a fence. No matter how much you worry about which way the cat will jump, you have no control over it.

Spiritual teachers never go into the future attaching emotionally to events that may or may not occur. Why, then, do we? Stress and the impact of stress hormones occur when we don't let go of past hurts and worry about events that have not yet happened. Remember the simple saying: "Right thoughts, right deeds, right actions." This is a path to inner peace.

Satguru Sivaya Subramuniyaswami, the founder of Kauai's Hindu Monastery, teaches that whenever you start to worry, ask yourself, "Am I all right?" Then declare, "I am all right, right now." When your mind drifts into worry, bring it back to the present moment. Use the mantra, "Present moment, only moment." Sit quietly and breathe in peace, breathe out worry. Every time you begin to worry or feel fear and anxiety, ask, "Am I all right?" Then again declare, "I am all right, right now." Each time you repeat this affirmation, you will feel positive and let go of fears and worries. Don't just say this affirmation; feel it to the very core of your being. Practice this simple yet powerful tool over and over again. "Am I all right?" I am all right, right now!

103. Remember Who You Are.

I was invited to Calgary, Alberta, to spend time with my spiritual teacher. After two days of meditation and prayer, I was asked by a friend to attend a Canada Day celebration. I knew there would be good food, loud music, and lots of alcohol. I was having some angst about going, and I expressed this to my teacher. He listened intently as I explained about not wanting to shift from such peaceful energy to a big party. I will never forget his response: "Mimi, remember who you are."

I have been asking myself that question ever since. Who are *you*? Many people believe that the Divine is outside of them. They identify with the physical body, which has clearly defined physical limitations. They believe their happiness is connected to owning things and acquiring material objects. Each purchase leads to wanting something more and brings worry that what they have will be lost. It is hard to be content and at peace. Connecting to your soul, which is part of the Divine, is not limited to a few groups or individuals—it exists within every human being. Just as a single drop of water still has all the properties of water, each of us has a spark of the Divine, totally intact and without any missing pieces. Remember, this is the ultimate goal of the spiritual path.

Stand in front of a mirror and ask a simple question:

"Who am I?"

If I change my hair color, am I not the same person? What if I change my name or my profession? Who am I?

Some answers might be:

I am a sister, brother, mother, father, husband, wife, aunt, uncle, friend.

I am a teacher, doctor, professor, caregiver, nurse.

I am a child of God, a spark of the Divine.

I am spirit in a physical body.

I am love, pure love.

Repeat this exercise over and over until you connect with the essence of who you really are.

104. Define Your State of Consciousness: Heaven or Hell?

Our feelings are many, but they are derived from two basic emotions: love and fear. All positive emotions—gratitude, joy, compassion, kindness—come from love. All negative emotions— anger, resentment, jealousy, envy, control—come from fear. As humans, we experience a full range of emotions throughout the day. Many of the negative emotions, as we have seen, are detrimental to our health.

Draw a line down the center of a piece of paper. Label the page "Emotions" and make two columns. List all the emotions you experience throughout the day. Put positive emotions on the left and negative emotions on the right. For example, hate is a high-energy negative emotion, while love is a high-energy positive emotion.

We all have a full range of emotions. When do you experience love, compassion, empathy, and forgiveness? Depression, anger, greed, and hatred? Where do you spend most of your day? Which emotions can you recognize and change? How do you want others to remember the way you make them feel?

Learn to be a passive observer of your day. Watch your thoughts and your behavior without judgment; just note where and how you spend your time. You will most likely find that during any given day, you travel an emotional road back and forth, from the heaven of positive emotions to the hell of negative emotions. How can you stay in the middle of the road? Or, better yet, be more on the side of love, gratefulness, compassion, and appreciation? Monitor your thoughts and actions. Before saying something negative, take a few deep breaths and ask your heart for a better answer. If your thoughts are negative, switch them to something that brings you happiness and joy. Break the cycle of negative thinking by consciously choosing your thoughts. Repeat your mantra or sacred word over and over again.

105. Let Your Light Shine—and See the Light in Others.

Alex Grey is an extraordinary contemporary artist who had an installation in New York City called the Chapel of Sacred Mirrors. The exhibit consists of 19 paintings and two etched mirrors that examine the body, mind, and spirit in astonishing detail. It begins with greater-than-life images of men and women with different skin colors, body sizes, and builds. As the exhibit progresses, the outer layers of skin coloring are slowly peeled away, revealing muscle, organs, bone, and lymphatics. The human energy system is depicted in amazing detail. Once the first layer of skin coloring is removed, the underlying muscle, bone, and organ systems reveal the unity of humanity as it becomes impossible to tell black from white, male from female. The last image is pure white light.

In many spiritual traditions, human beings are referred to as beams of light. In Christianity, we speak about the light of Christ, and in the yogic tradition, we say *namaste*, which translates to "the light in me greets the light in you." In the words of His Holiness the Dalai Lama, "We have 7.5 billion light beings living on the planet." So in essence, we all are beams of light.

This concept is no surprise to quantum physicists, who recognize light as frequency and vibration. Every object, including human beings, vibrates at a particular frequency, some higher, some lower. But what would happen if, as Alex Grey's paintings suggest, we pull off the outer layers of difference and see each other as radiant beams of light? Would we be more tolerant and less judgmental?

I remember a unity minister telling the story of a monastery in China. The monks, in fear that their sacred statue of Buddha would be destroyed, hid the pure gold statue under layers and layers of mud. Generations of monks later, a golden light was noted shining through the mud covering. The monks began to chip away at the mud to reveal a pure golden statue of Buddha. Sometimes we are like that statue. Covered in layers of hurt and pain, we sometimes find it difficult to recognize our own light or see the light in others. But just like the golden Buddha, your light is definitely present.

In the Kundalini yoga tradition, classes close with the mantra *sat nam*, which means "I am truth, truth is my identity." When you pull back your fear, judgment, resentment, and other emotions that never serve your highest good, your light begins to shine. When you replace these emotions and negative thoughts with compassion, you begin to see the light in others.

Find a simple exercise to connect with your spirit or higher self. Try spending more time in nature by walking through a forest or open field or sitting at the beach and listening to the waves.

Begin your day by sitting quietly in meditation and use your mantra or sacred word to anchor your thoughts. Try to meditate for 20 minutes; when your mind begins to wander, mentally repeat your sacred word or mantra to bring your thoughts back to the present moment. Listen to sacred music or chants and let the vibration of the music connect with your spirit. Don't worry about the words; just let the music carry you to a place of inner peace.

106. Open Your Heart. Love Is Always the Answer.

When we fall in love, we feel inspired and excited about everything in our lives. No matter how old we are, we feel happy, light, and full of energy. We sail through challenges with a one-day-at-a-time attitude, and we see the good in everything.

When we lose love, we feel heavy and overwhelmed. Somehow everything seems more stressful and chaotic.

Remember, there are all kinds of love. Unconditional love is what we feel for our babies, our grandchildren, and our pets. We look at them and hold them with love in our hearts and hands. We feel joy, and our heart sings. Can you extend unconditional love to those around you? Can you extend unconditional love to yourself?

Try this exercise to open your heart and awaken the power of love!

- Close your eyes and imagine roots growing from the soles of your feet and attaching deep into the earth's core.

- Slowly pull the energy up from the earth up into your ankles, knees, and hips.

- Bring the earth's energy up into your spine and slowly into your heart center.

- Imagine your heart center as a beam of golden light that begins to grow and expand. Let the light run down your arms to the center of your palms. Let the

light expand from your heart and surround your
body, enfolding you with love and compassion. Now,
imagine the light from your heart expanding to fill
the room, the building, your neighborhood, and
the planet.

• You are now in your heart's center, and you are
the essence of love. From this space, you touch
everything and everyone with the hands of love.
Send love to yourself, your loved ones, those in
need, and the planet. Remain in this sacred space
for as long as you feel comfortable, and then slowly
imagine coming back into your body.

107. Manifest Your Reality and Bring Your Dreams to Fruition.

When I refer patients for Healing Touch treatments, it is usually because they need more than conventional medicine can
offer. Maggie was a perfect example. She was 74 years old, a widow,
and a practicing Catholic, and she had been my patient since I
placed a simple stent in her artery in the 1990s.

Maggie came to the emergency room three or four times per
month with various complaints, yet all her tests consistently came
back normal. She frequently complained about chest pain, but
there was no physical explanation.

With no tangible reason for her health challenges, I suggested
we explore a different approach. She was lonely, low on money,
and under enormous stress since the death of her husband. Her
older daughter was in and out of jail for drug abuse and burglary.
It was clear to me that Maggie had a broken heart; the death of her
husband and her daughter's drug abuse had left her with pain and
disappointment. I referred her to Rauni King for a Healing Touch
treatment in the hope that it would decrease her stress and alleviate her suffering.

During her treatment, Maggie mentioned that she was lonely. She wanted someone to share her life with. Rauni suggested to Maggie that she pray to find the right partner, to which she immediately responded, "I feel unfaithful to my husband."

"Nonsense," Rauni said. "Pray to your deceased husband and ask him to help you."

Maggie followed Rauni's advice. Each night for the next week, she lit a candle and asked her husband to help her find the perfect companion. She prayed for guidance and was clear to the universe on whom and what she wanted.

Maggie was shocked when, approximately two weeks later, there was a surprise knock on her front door. It was her neighbor, a successful businessman, inviting her out to dinner. That dinner turned into a 15-year marriage, a beautiful home, financial security, and a loving relationship. Maggie manifested the love of her life, and her trips to the emergency room became a joke about the past.

108. Set Your Intention On the Life You Want.

The native priests of Hawaii had it right: Our thoughts are alive. They have energy. What we think about expands into the universe, and the universe takes clear messages—we call them intentions—and reflects them back to us. When we set our intentions clearly, we give the universe the direction it needs to make them reality. But we also must be realistic. Let's face it; I will never be a professional boxer.

Where to start? Think about something you know you really want. Is it a new apartment, a new home, financial security, or a trusting relationship? Next, we will practice what yoga master Paramahansa Yogananda calls the law of abundance. This law implies that the Cosmic Creator is more than willing to bestow blessings on each and every one of us; there is an unlimited supply of health, happiness, and prosperity.

Once you connect with this abundant universal energy, you are that much closer to your own dream of manifesting blessings in your life.

Determine what it is you want, in your life, at this moment. Visualize how you want your life to look. Where would you be living, and with whom? Would there be a garden in your yard? A place to practice yoga or Tai Chi? A sacred space for meditation? It could be that simple. Ask yourself what would make you most happy and content: what would make you feel healthy and alive. Would it be a less stressful job or a more loving relationship?

Set aside time each day for prayer or meditation. Place your mind in a state of relaxation and contemplation. You may even start by repeating your mantra or sacred word using a strand of 108 beads, from one to 108—my last and most precious pearl of wisdom. Calm your mind and relax your body through meditation, breath work, or mantra repetition. Once you are in a calm and peaceful state, remain there, quiet and composed, focused on your intentions. Be exact and definite in your requests. See the things you desire in your mind. Envision yourself in your new home or working happily at your new job. Be very, very clear in your mind about the feeling this brings you. Next, imagine yourself living and experiencing your manifestation as if it has already happened. Use your mind to see your desire as if you are living it. Don't just see it, feel it! The trick is to feel it as if you are living it. Feel yourself in your new environment, at your new job, or with your new partner. It is important to feel the way you would feel if you were living in your dream in the present moment. Put the words to manifest your intentions in present terms. Your words have energy. For example, you could say, "I am living in a cottage with a beautiful yard" or "I am working with animals at a job I love." Be very specific.

There is only thing left to do: Thank the universe in advance for bringing your request to fruition. It is already done.

• ● •

AFTERWORD

Reclaiming Our Health: Body, Mind, and Spirit

The energy of the mala can be truly transformational. As we count our breath and our blessings, it gives us something both physical and spiritual to hold on to. Just as each of the 108 beads takes us into deeper reflection and guides us from separation to unity, each of the 108 pearls outlined in this book serves as a guide to awaken our healing potential. With each step we take, we get closer to achieving our best possible selves—healthy and thriving, nourishing what matters most. We understand that our thoughts and our habits affect not only our own lives but also the world in which we live. To inspire greater health in our lives is to embrace a greater purpose.

With each pearl of wisdom in this book, I've invited you to look after the planet, to care for those around you, and to nourish your own body and soul with knowledge, love, and patience. It is my hope that you now know yourself better, from your body composition and vital stats, to the way you eat and respond to stress, to your emotional and spiritual well-being. Through this discovery, perhaps you have begun to adopt new habits and ways of thinking that enhance your health and lead to transformation. Know that each choice you make, each word you utter, and each thought you think has the opportunity to heal body, mind, and spirit.

While many acknowledge the importance of the health of body and mind, do not forget this crucial aspect of health—the spirit. Spiritual teachers often call it the Divine spark, or "true self." This recognition of the Divine spark and self as one can be realized or uncovered by each and every individual. Alone we represent one spark of the Divine, but each individual spark comes from the main source, linking us together in a constant urging to return home to spirit. Just like each drop within the ocean contains all the components of water, we each contain all the components of the Divine: love, compassion, and goodness.

Origen, a third-century Greek theologian of the Christian Church, referred to this spark of love and goodness as a seed that has been planted by God in the consciousness of all individuals. As an apple seed grows to bear apples, a God seed grows to bear Divine fruit, which is love and compassion for all people and our planet. All it needs to grow is a gardener who is willing to go within, to occasionally leave the created world and seek the uncreated. You are that gardener.

In a small town more than 700 years ago, Meister Eckhart said: "I have spoken at times of a light in the soul, a light that is uncreated and uncreatable . . . to the extent that we can deny ourselves and turn away from created things, we shall find our unity and blessing in the little spark in the soul, which neither space nor time touches." Yet our human experience, filled with ego, covers up this jewel within and leads us on a journey of seeking happiness from outside sources. Eventually, if we are lucky, the toys of materialism, larger homes, and bigger cars no longer satisfy our needs and we begin to ask the profound question: "Is that all there is?" Meister Eckert challenges us to turn away from the manmade and materialistic. He suggests we will find our unity and blessing "in the little spark in the soul."

Spiritual teachers consider this recognition of the unity of all life to be our highest goal and one of the main reasons for our human birth. Yogi Bajan said, "The energy of the universe is yours. It is your birthright. Just claim it." Once we recognize the Divine within ourselves, we recognize that we are connected to all living creatures. This connection transforms our very existence because once we know there is no difference between you and me; instead, we see the interconnectedness and unity of all aspects of life.

This connection is what accounts for the joy that we receive in service—what we do for others we indeed do for ourselves. It also speaks to our connection to the planet as a vital component of our web of life. This philosophy has been taught for centuries by many spiritual teachers and is not unique to one religious or spiritual tradition. Jesus referred to this recognition when he said "the kingdom of Heaven is within." In Judaism, the presence of God, *Shekinah*, is found within all of creation.

Once we have an awareness of this spark of goodness in all life forms, everything changes. Our very actions become a reflection of this insight. We become less interested in personal fortune and the need to accumulate material items. We become more compassionate and see through the eyes of love. No matter what challenges we have in our lives, no matter what mistakes we have made, the spark of love and goodness is within each and every one of us. There is no need to look outward for this goodness, no place to buy it—it is there for us always.

When it comes down to it, most of us desire the same things: love, happiness, a sense of purpose, joy, and inner peace. It's in the ways we choose to achieve these things that vary. But almost as soon as we achieve whatever we thought we desired—moving into that bigger house, driving away in that expensive car—we are looking for our next pleasure. We never have enough when we are looking in all the wrong places. Take a moment to truly reflect on the words of the song "Amazing Grace": "I once was lost but now am found, was blind but now I see."

So are you willing to look within? This is not an easy question. It requires that we practice right thoughts and right actions. We need to change how we think and act, and how we see the world. It requires going on a journey from *me* to *we*. We have the resources to feed, clothe, house, and care for all people and our planet. But are we making the *right* choices? Only through the lens of love do we stand the chance of saving ourselves, our community, our nation, and the planet.

• ● •

APPENDIX A

The Medical Symptom/Toxicity Questionnaire

The Toxicity and Symptom Screening Questionnaire identifies symptoms that help to identify the underlying causes of illness, and helps you track your progress over time. The first time you complete this questionnaire, rate each of the following symptoms based upon your health profile for the past 30 days. After your first time, record your symptoms for the last 48 hours *only*.

POINT SCALE: Assign yourself points according to the severity and frequency with which you experience symptoms:

0 = Never, or almost never, have the symptom
1 = Occasionally have the symptom, effect is not severe
2 = Occasionally have the syptom, effect is severe
3 = Frequently have the symptom, effect is not severe
4 = Frequently have the symptom, effect is severe

KEY TO QUESTIONNAIRE: Add individual scores, and then total each group. Add each group score for your grand total.

Optimal: <10 • Mild Toxicity: 10–50 • Moderate Toxicity: 50–100 • Severe Toxicity: 100+

Grand Total: _____

DIGESTIVE TRACT

_____ Nausea or vomiting

_____ Diarrhea

_____ Constipation

_____ Bloated feeling

_____ Belching or passing gas

_____ Heartburn

_____ Intestinal/stomach pain

Total: _____

EARS

_____ Itchy ears

_____ Earaches, ear infections

_____ Drainage from ear

_____ Ringing in ears, hearing loss

Total: _____

EMOTIONS

_____ Mood swings

_____ Anxiety, fear, or nervousness

_____ Anger, irritability,
or aggressiveness

_____ Depression

Total: _____

ENERGY/ACTIVITY

_____ Fatigue, sluggishness

_____ Apathy, lethargy

_____ Hyperactivity

_____ Restlessness

Total: _____

EYES

_____ Watery or itchy eyes

_____ Swollen, reddened,
or sticky eyelids

_____ Bags or dark circles under eyes

_____ Blurred or tunnel vision (does not

_____ include near- or far-sightedness)

Total: _____

HEAD

_____ Headaches

_____ Faintness

_____ Dizziness

_____ Insomnia

Total: _____

HEART

_____ Irregular or skipped heartbeat

_____ Rapid or pounding heartbeat

_____ Chest pain

Total: _____

JOINTS/MUSCLES

_____ Pain or aches in joints

_____ Arthritis

_____ Stiffness or limitation
of movement

_____ Pain or aches in muscles

_____ Feeling of weakness or tiredness

Total: _____

LUNGS

_____ Chest congestion

_____ Asthma, bronchitis

_____ Shortness of breath

_____ Difficulty breathing

Total: _____

MIND

_____ Poor memory

_____ Confusion, poor comprehension

_____ Poor physical coordination

_____ Difficulty in making decisions

_____ Stuttering or stammering

_____ Slurred speech

_____ Learning disabilities

Total: _____

MOUTH/THROAT

_____ Chronic cough

_____ Gagging, frequent need to clear
throat

_____ Sore throat, hoarseness,
loss of voice

_____ Swollen or discolored tongue,
gum, and/or lips

_____ Canker sores

Total: _____

NOSE

_____ Stuffy nose

_____ Sinus problems

_____ Hay fever

_____ Sneezing attacks

_____ Excessive mucus formation

Total: _____

SKIN

_____ Acne

_____ Hives, rashes, or dry skin

_____ Hair loss

_____ Flushing, hot flushes

_____ Excessive sweating

Total: _____

WEIGHT

_____ Binge eating or drinking

_____ Cravings for certain foods

_____ Being overweight

_____ Being underweight

_____ Compulsive eating

_____ Water retention

Total: _____

OTHER

_____ Frequent illness

_____ Frequent or urgent urination

_____ Genital itching or discharge

Total: _____

APPENDIX B

Guide to the Elimination Diet

Many people notice that they feel bad after eating. Others note that they have fatigue, gas, bloating, arthritic pain, or brain fog. Sometimes it is easy to associate the food with the reaction, and sometimes it isn't. Reasons for confusion include food combinations, the quantity consumed, and the total "load" of reactive foods, antibodies, and toxins in the body. To address the problem, you may follow a dietary program designed to clear the body of foods and chemicals that you may be allergic or sensitive to and then experimentally test foods one at a time.

By first eliminating known or suspected foods, you allow your body's detoxification machinery, which may be overburdened or compromised, to recover and begin to function efficiently again. This also allows the immune system to "quiet down" and reduce the production of antibodies to foods, thereby reducing inflammation.

I strongly suggest that you try the elimination diet if you have a high score on the Medical Symptom/Toxicity Questionnaire that I use in my practice (see Appendix A) or have arthritis, mental fogginess, fatigue, skin rashes, or gastrointestinal symptoms.

The Setup

There are two phases to this diet: a four-week elimination phase and a two-to-four-week challenge phase.

Elimination Phase

During this four-week phase, you remove certain foods from your diet. You can eliminate one or more food categories at a time. I suggest that if you are very symptomatic, you eliminate *all* of the most common food irritants—dairy, gluten, corn, soy, tree nuts, citrus, and egg. Some people may also need to eliminate shellfish.

To determine which foods to eliminate, start with the most common allergens. Alternatively, you might ask your doctor to order blood tests or get clues from your nutrition diary. For example, people frequently feel that they can't live without certain foods, such as dairy or wheat. The food category you crave the most is commonly the offending one.

Be sure to eliminate not only the food itself but also any other foods that may include that ingredient. Dairy, for example, includes all milk, cream, cheese, cottage cheese, yogurt, ice cream, frozen yogurt, and butter. It even includes milk chocolate. If a food contains butter or whey as an ingredient, it's also off-limits.

If you are eliminating gluten, remember that it is in wheat, spelt, rye, barley, malt, and cereals. Condiments such as ketchup, mayonnaise, and mustard all contain vinegar that frequently comes from wheat or corn and so will contain trace amounts of gluten. You have to read the labels carefully. You will be surprised how many foods contain wheat, soy, or corn. If you are sensitive to oats, avoid them unless the package specifies they are gluten-free.

Eliminate all foods from the chosen category or categories for two weeks. If your symptoms improve during the four-week period, you know you have a sensitivity to one or more of the eliminated food or category of foods. Now the question becomes, which one(s)? To find out, you carefully add foods back into your diet, one at a time, to see which may trigger symptoms.

For example, for one day, eat some dairy. Then wait 48 hours for your body to respond. If your symptoms return, you know that dairy is a culprit. Now pick another category, such as gluten. Eat gluten-containing products for one day, and then wait for your body to respond. Keep a journal of how you feel.

Most often, individuals on the elimination diet report increased energy, mental alertness, decrease in muscle or joint pain, and a general sense of improved well-being. Many people lose weight. However, some people report some initial reactions to the diet, especially in the first week. This can include caffeine withdrawal headaches and other "Herxheimer-type" reactions. These are hangover-like symptoms as the body metabolizes and detoxifies accumulated toxins. Symptoms you may experience in the first week can include changes in sleep patterns, lightheadedness, headaches, joint or muscle stiffness, and changes in gastrointestinal function. If this occurs, try to keep going. Your body will detoxify, and you will begin to feel better. Your doctor will want to see you at the end of the month to evaluate the changes in your health. Although, dairy gluten, soy, corn, and egg are the most common allergens, some individuals are sensitive to citrus, shellfish, and tree nuts.

Challenge Phase

During the challenge phase, foods are systematically added back into the diet and careful notes are made about the appearance of any symptoms. Again, track your symptoms in your food journal. You will introduce a new food every 48 hours, assuming you feel well. Here's the general process: select the food you want to challenge. Eat the test food at least twice a day and in a fairly large amount. Often, an offending food will provoke symptoms quickly—within 10 minutes to 12 hours. Signs to look for include: headache, itching, bloating, nausea, dizziness, fatigue, diarrhea, indigestion, anal itching, sleepiness 30 minutes after a meal, flushing, or rapid heartbeat. Sometimes you won't notice symptoms until the next morning: puffy eyes, can't get out of bed, brain-fog, more typing errors than usual. If you are unsure, take the food back out of your diet for at least one week and try it again. Be sure to test foods in a pure form: for example, test milk or cheese or wheat but not macaroni and cheese that contains milk, cheese, *and* wheat!

Tips for the Elimination Diet

- If you have symptoms after eating some foods, remember, it is not a death sentence! Your experience during the elimination diet is *information*, and with it, you are empowered to choose what you want to eat and how you want to feel. Sometimes, sharing a piece of birthday cake with someone special is completely worth gas, bloating, and baggy eyes!

- People whose food sensitivities are related to intestinal permeability or inflammation may be able to incorporate small amounts of allergenic foods in four to six months. People who have autoimmune cross-reactions to foods should minimize exposure their whole lives.

- Ideally, you eliminate *all* sources of potentially allergenic foods. This means that you must read labels carefully! However, life happens—people forget to tell you what ingredients they used, waiters are wrong, and so on. Don't sweat it—do the best you can. If you are exposed to *a lot* of allergens, you may want to extend the elimination phase a little longer. Eat a wide variety of foods, and do not try to restrict your calorie intake. Use the opportunity to try new ingredients and venture into new ethnic restaurants; this is a journey of self-exploration and discovery!

- Avoid any foods that you know or believe you may be sensitive to, even if they are on the "allowed" list.

- Plan your meals. Eat regular meals. Eat simply. Cook simply.

- Cook extra chicken, sweet potatoes, rice, and beans, etc., that can be reheated for snacking or another meal.

- Get in the habit of using leftovers for the next day's meal or part of a meal—e.g., leftover broiled salmon and broccoli from dinner as part of a large salad for lunch the next day.

- The first two to three days are the hardest. It's important to go shopping for foods you are allowed to have.

- Be sure to snack to keep your blood sugar levels normal and stable. Carry food with you when you leave the house. That way, you will have what you are allowed and not be tempted to stray off the plan.

- Try to eat *at least* three servings of fresh vegetables each day. Choose at least one serving of dark green or orange vegetables (carrot, broccoli, winter squash) and one raw vegetable each day. Vary your selections.

- Buy organic produce when possible. Select fresh foods whenever you can. If possible, choose organically grown fruits and vegetables to reduce your exposure to synthetic pesticides and chemical residues. Wash fruits and vegetables thoroughly.

- If you are consuming coffee or other caffeine-containing beverages on a regular basis, slowly reduce your caffeine intake rather than abruptly stop it; this will prevent caffeine-withdrawal headaches. For instance, try drinking half decaf/half regular coffee for a few days, then slowly reduce the total amount of coffee.

- If you are a vegetarian, consume more beans and rice, quinoa, seeds, nuts, amaranth, teff, millet, and buckwheat.

- If you select animal sources of protein, look for free-range or organically raised chicken, turkey, or lamb. Cold-water fish (e.g., salmon, sardines, mackerel, and halibut) is an excellent source of protein and omega-3 essential fatty acids. To select low-mercury, sustainable fish, check out www.seafoodwatch.org or download the Seafood Watch mobile app.

- During this time, you may want to augment your diet with an organic, freeze-dried, powdered greens and protein supplement. (We like Greens First.) Hemp and pea protein are great, and few people are allergic to these foods.

- Remember to drink at least two quarts of filtered water each day. If you hate plain water, add trace mineral drops, make herbal iced tea, or consider bubbly water.

- Consider taking a break from strenuous exercise to allow the body to heal more effectively without the additional burden imposed by exercise. This is a great time for yoga, walking, and hiking. Adequate rest and stress reduction is also important to the success of this program.

If you find no improvement within four to six weeks, it is possible that you do not have any food allergies. It is also possible that you have food allergies, but there another factor is complicating the picture, and you'll need to consult with your doctor.

Elimination Diet Guidelines

Foods to Include	Foods to Exclude
Whole, low-sugar fruits and unsweetened juices	High-sugar fruits such as oranges; fruit juices with added sugar
Dairy alternatives such as rice, almond, hemp, coconut milk	Dairy made with cow's milk, including cheese, cottage cheese, cream, yogurt, butter, ice cream, and frozen yogurt; nondairy creamers
Nongluten grains and starch, including rice (all types), millet, quinoa, amaranth, teff, tapioca, buckwheat, potato flour (Note that some gluten-free grains have a high glycemic load. If you are trying to lose weight, minimize carbohydrates.)	Grains with gluten, wheat, corn, barley, spelt, rye, triticale, oat
Animal protein: fresh or water-packed canned fish, wild game, lamb, duck, organic chicken and turkey, and organic, free-range eggs	Animal protein: pork, beef/veal, sausage, cold cuts, canned meats, frankfurters, shellfish
Vegetable protein: split peas, lentils, mung beans, and legumes of all kinds (black, white, Northern, cannellini, and pinto beans; fresh and frozen peas)	Soybean products (soy sauce, soybean oil in processed foods, tempeh, tofu, soy milk, soy yogurt, textured vegetable protein)
Nuts and seeds, including coconut, pine nuts, flaxseed, walnuts; sesame, pumpkin, and sunflower seeds, hazelnuts, pecans, almonds, cashews; nut and seed butters (Some individuals have nut sensitivities. If you cannot find the source of your symptoms, consider the elimination of all nuts except pine nuts and coconut.)	Peanuts and peanut butter
Vegetables: all raw, steamed, sautéed, juiced, or roasted (except corn) (If you have arthritis, avoid nightshades: tomatoes, potatoes, eggplants, peppers, paprika, salsa, chili peppers, cayenne, chili powder.)	Corn and creamed vegetables.

Foods to Include	Foods to Exclude
Oils: cold pressed olive, ghee, oils from avocado, grapeseed, coconut, organic butter	Nonorganic butter, margarine, shortening, processed oils (most canola, soy, vegetable, safflower oils), processed salad dressings, mayonnaise, and spreads
Drinks: filtered or distilled water, decaffeinated herbal teas, seltzer, mineral water	Drinks: alcohol, coffee, caffeinated beverages, soft drinks
Sweets (sparingly): Manuka honey, coconut crystals; dark chocolate with >60-70% cacao (dairy free)	Refined white and brown sugar, high-fructose corn syrup, evaporated cane juice, agave nectar
Condiments: vinegar and all spices, including salt, pepper, basil, carob, cinnamon, cumin, dill, garlic, ginger, mustard, oregano, parsley, rosemary, tarragon, thyme, turmeric	Processed and high-sugar condiments, including ketchup, relish, chutney, soy sauce, barbecue sauce, and teriyaki

Things to Watch for:

- Corn starch in baking powder and any processed foods

- Corn syrup in beverages and processed foods

- Breads advertised as gluten-free may contain oats, spelt, kamut, rye

- Many amaranth and millet flake cereals have oats or corn

- Many canned tunas contain textured vegetable protein, which is from soy; look for low-salt versions, which tend to be pure tuna with no fillers

- Buckwheat is not wheat and can be eaten, but check for other grains in premixed flours

Substitutions and Alternatives

Cow's milk	Rice, hemp, coconut, almond, or homemade nut milk (1/2 cup raw nuts or seeds with 1 cup water, blended until smooth; or soaked and pressed)
Cheese	Rice and almond brands: read labels and look for casein-free brands. Nutritional yeast adds a similar richness
Eggs (for baking)	Egg replacer (EnergE brand is one. Note that these are not the same as egg substitutes, which may still contain eggs). Applesauce, mashed banana. Or blend 1 tablespoon of flaxseed in blender with 1/4 cup water and allow to thicken
Peanut butter	Nut butters made from almonds, cashews, macadamia, walnut, pumpkin, hazelnut, or sesame (tahini)
Breading	Grind any allowable rice cracker or nuts and use as breading
Ice cream	Coconut or rice ice cream (vanilla), frozen bars of 100% fruit juice, berry sorbets
Soda	Seltzer and juice, water, diluted juice
Jams	100% all-fruit jams (read label carefully)
Sugar	Brown rice syrup; stevia, maple syrup, honey; fruit juice concentrate (Mystic Lake Dairy or Wax Orchard, for example)
Pasta	Gluten-free pastas (quinoa, rice, buckwheat, buckwheat, spinach, lentil), buckwheat udon noodles, cellophane noodles made from bean threads, shirataki noodles made from yam
Wheat bread	Rice cakes, rice crackers, nut crackers, gluten-free breads, nonwheat tortillas. (Remember that oats, spelt, and rye contain gluten, so read labels carefully on products labeled "multigrain.")
Wheat cereals	Gluten-free cereals, puffed rice, puffed millet, cream of rice, gluten-free hot cereal
Wheat flour	Rice, quinoa, amaranth, millet, teff, arrowroot; nut and seed flours. Use in combination (at least 3) to replace the full amount of wheat flour and add 1/2 teaspoon xanthan gum per cup

Elimination Diet Shopping List

Fruits

Apples, applesauce
Apricots (fresh)
Bananas
Blackberries
Blueberries
Cantaloupe
Cherries
Coconut
Figs (fresh)
Grapefruit
Huckleberries
Kiwi
Kumquat
Lemon, lime
Loganberries
Mangos
Melons
Mulberries
Nectarines
Papayas
Peaches
Pears
Prunes
Raspberries
Strawberries

Vegetables*

Artichoke
Asparagus
Avocado
Bamboo shoots
Beets and beet tops
Bok choy
Broccoflower
Broccoli
Brussels sprouts
Cabbage
Bell peppers
Carrots
Cauliflower
Celery
Chives
Cucumber
Dandelion greens
Eggplant
Endive
Kale
Kohlrabi
Leeks
Lettuce: red leaf
  or
  green leaf,
  or Chinese
Mushroom
Okra
Onions

Parsley
Potato
Radicchio
  (red leaf chicory)
Sea vegetables:
  seaweed, kelp
Snow peas
Spinach
Squash
Sweet potatoes
Swiss chard
Tomato
Watercress
Yams
Zucchini

*If you have arthritis,
avoid nightshades,
which are denoted by
italics.

Herbs, Spices, and Extracts

Any and all!
  Particularly
  rosemary, basil,
  oregano, turmeric,
  saffron, garlic, and
  cinnamon

Gluten-Free Grains and Breads

Amaranth

Breads, any gluten-free varieties

Buckwheat

Millet

Quinoa

Rice: brown, white, wild Teff

Cereals and Pasta

Buckwheat noodles

Cream of rice

Puffed rice

Puffed millet

Quinoa flakes

Rice pasta

Rice crackers/rice cakes

Dairy Substitutes

Almond milk

Coconut milk

Hemp milk

Rice milk

Oils

Coconut

Flax

Ghee

Olive

Animal Protein

Fresh ocean fish (e.g., Pacific salmon, halibut, haddock, cod, sole, pollock, tuna, mahi-mahi.

Lamb

Poultry: free-range chicken, turkey, duck

Water-packed canned tuna (watch for added protein from soy)

Wild game

Nuts

Any nut but peanut

Vinegars

Apple Cider

Balsamic

Red wine

Rice

Tarragon

Ume plum

Sweeteners

Agave nectar

Coconut crystals (preferred)

Fruit sweetener (100% juice concentrate)

Manuka honey

Molasses

Rice syrup

Stevia

Condiments

Mustard (made with apple cider vinegar)

Beverages

Fruit or vegetable juices, unsweetened (dilute with water before drinking)

Herbal tea (noncaffeinated)

Mineral water

Spring water

Baking Supplies

Arrowroot /xanthan gum

Baking soda

Flours: rice, teff, quinoa, millet, tapioca, amaranth, potato, tapioca

Pure vanilla extract

Elimination Diet Menu Ideas

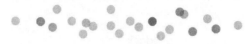

Here are some ideas to stimulate your own creativity:

Breakfast: Consider eating "dinner" foods—there's no reason not to enjoy a savory soup in the morning! Feel free to add protein powder drinks, leftover chicken, fish, and such to your breakfast menu.

- Cooked whole grain (brown rice, buckwheat, teff, or quinoa) served with fresh or frozen fruit. You can add a bit of coconut oil or flakes, ghee, manuka honey, and/or cinnamon. To boost protein, mix in nuts or have a protein-powder drink. Chia seeds add extra omega-3.

- Home-fried potatoes: Cut onions, peppers (a nightshade), broccoli, mushrooms, and other vegetables of your choice into small pieces and sauté in coconut oil or ghee. Cut prebaked potatoes (be aware that potatoes are nightshades and high on the glycemic index) into cubes and add to vegetables. Add salt, pepper, herbs, and spices such as rosemary and turmeric.

- "Fried" brown rice: Use the recipe above, substituting brown rice for the potatoes to decrease glycemic load.

- Toasted rice or lentil flax bread with coconut oil or ghee. Spread it with 100 percent fruit jam, or apple or pear butter. Add fresh fruit, herbal tea.

- Fruit smoothie: Blend rice or coconut milk with fruit such as organic berries, bananas, pears, pineapple, mango, or papaya. Add fish oil as desired. Add fiber to your smoothies with gluten-free oats, hemp, flax, chia, or psyllium seeds as desired. Not only does fiber improve digestion and lower cholesterol and blood sugar, it also helps you feel more satiated.

- Brown-rice pancakes topped with apple butter, apple sauce, or sautéed apples.

- Gluten-free oatmeal or amaranth or other gluten-free cereal (read label carefully) with fresh fruit (bananas, berries, pears, apples, etc.) and rice or coconut milk.

- Half a cantaloupe filled with blueberries, or half a papaya with unsweetened coconut yogurt.

Lunch or Dinner:

- Large salad with baked chicken or fish.

- Baked salmon plus steamed or oven-roasted vegetables with cooked quinoa or baked sweet potato or quinoa salad. Can also add a salad with vinaigrette dressing.

- Fruit salad with coconut or pine nuts. Serve with protein and rice crackers.

- Broiled or poached halibut, baked winter squash sprinkled with cinnamon and ghee, mixed green salad with vinaigrette dressing, and mocha rice squares and fruit for dessert.

- Brown rice and grilled chicken, steamed greens, baked potato or sweet potato.

- Halibut salad: Mixed greens of your choice, leftover halibut cut into chunks, vinaigrette dressing. Serve with baked potato with ghee.

- Chicken breast sprinkled with garlic powder and tarragon, steamed asparagus or broccoli, brown or wild rice or kasha, ghee or olive oil.

- Quinoa with lentil or vegetable soup.

- Quinoa salad with leftover chicken or fish.

- Quinoa salad with kale and bean soup.

- Broiled fresh tuna steak topped with herbs, brown-rice pasta with olive oil and fresh tomato sauce, steamed kale or collard greens tossed with olive oil and garlic and vinegar, mixed greens salad with vinaigrette dressing. Fruit for dessert.

- Tuna salad: Canned tuna mixed with vinaigrette or eggless mayonnaise, fresh fruit.

- Roast organic turkey breast or broiled bean burger, brown or wild rice, steamed vegetable, salad with vinaigrette. Baked apple or poached pear.

- Turkey salad: Leftover turkey breast, mixed greens, other fresh vegetables, lemon or oil and vinegar, rice crackers, fresh fruit or cup of soup.

- Brown-rice pasta primavera (vegetables added to pasta), mixed greens salad with vinaigrette, rice pudding topped with berries.

Snacks:

- Baby carrots and cucumbers with baba ganouj or hummus.

- Snap peas

- Fennel

- Half a pint of fresh organic berries

- Vegetables dipped into guacamole (jicama is especially good)

- Baked apple

- Poached pear

- Fresh-squeezed vegetable juice (great option when out and about)

- Fresh fruit

- Crunchy veggie sticks: carrots, cucumbers, sweet peppers (nightshade), celery, jicama

- Papaya with organic plain yogurt

- Baked sweet potato with plain yogurt

• ● •

APPENDIX C

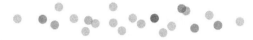

Mediterranean Diet Test

The following 14-point Mediterranean diet score was used in the Prevención con Dieta Mediterránea (PREDIMED) trial, which was a randomized trial to assess the role of the Mediterranean diet in preventing heart disease. It is a good benchmark for heart-healthy eating. Give yourself one point for each criterion that you meet. Ideally, your total score should be 9 or higher.

Questions	Criteria
1. Do you use olive oil as a main culinary fat?	Yes
2. How much olive oil do you consume a day (including oil used for frying, salads and out-of-house meals)?	≥4 tbsp
3. How many vegetable servings do you have a day? (1 serving = 200g [consider side dishes as half a serving])	≥2 (≥1 portion raw or as a salad)
4. How many fruit units (including natural fruit juices) do you eat a day?	≥3
5. How many servings of red meat, hamburger or meat products (ham, sausage, etc.) do you eat a day? (1 serving = 100–150g)	<1
6. How many servings of butter, margarine or cream do you have a day? (1 serving = 12 g)	<1
7. How many sweet or carbonated beverages do you drink a day?	<1
8. How many glasses of wine do you drink a week?	≥7 glasses*

9. How many servings of legumes do you eat a week? (1 serving = 150g)	≥3
10. How many servings of fish or shellfish do you eat a week? (1 serving = 100–150g of fish or 4–5 units or 200g of shellfish)	≥3
11. How many times per week do you consume commercial sweets or pastries (not homemade), such as cakes, cookies, biscuits or custard?	<3
12. How many servings of nuts (including peanuts) do you consume per week? (1 serving = 30g)	≥3
13. Do you preferentially choose chicken, turkey or rabbit meat instead of veal, pork, hamburger or sausage?	Yes**
14. How many times a week do you eat vegetables, pasta, rice or other dishes seasoned with sofrito (sauce made with tomato and onion, leek or garlic and simmered with olive oil)?	≥2
Total Score:	

*Be careful how you interpret the alcohol question. New guidelines recommend a maximum of one drink per day for men and a maximum of four drinks per week for women. The body sees alcohol as sugar and is packed with calories.

**The consumption of animal products has many undesirable side effects. Every time you consider eating an animal product, you must ask yourself what the animal ate. For example, milk from a cow that is treated with steroids and hormones is not desirable. Processed foods and animals farmed and raised on feedlots such as those in the United States are not part of the traditional Mediterranean diet.

• ● •

APPENDIX D

Glycemic Index and Glycemic Load

Food	Glycemic Index	Serving Size	Net Carbs	Glycemic Load
Bean sprouts	25	1 cup (104g)	4	1
Peanuts	14	4 oz (113g)	15	2
Carrots	47	1 large (72g)	5	2
Grapefruit	25	1/2 large (166g)	11	3
Apples	38	1 medium (138g)	16	6
Oranges	48	1 medium (131g)	12	6
Popcorn	72	2 cups (16g)	10	7
Sugar (sucrose)	68	1 tbsp (12g)	12	8
Watermelon	72	1 cup (154g)	11	8
Honey	55	1 tbsp (21g)	17	9
Ice cream	61	1 cup (72g)	16	10
White bread	70	1 slice (30g)	14	10
Oatmeal	58	1 cup (234g)	21	12
Bananas	52	1 large (136g)	27	14
Low-fat yogurt	33	1 cup (245g)	47	16
Spaghetti	42	1 cup (140g)	38	16
Raisins	64	1 small box (43g)	32	20
Brown rice	55	1 cup (195g)	42	23
Baked potato	85	1 medium (173g)	33	28
Potato chips	54	4 oz (114g)	55	30
Macaroni and cheese	64	1 serving (166g)	47	30
White rice	64	1 cup (186g)	52	33
Snickers Bar	55	1 bar (113g)	64	35
Glucose	100	(50g)	50	50

To make better choices, select most of your food from the left column in the following food categories.

Breads

Low GI: 55 or less (good choice)	Moderate GI: 56–69	higher (avoid/limit)
100% whole-grain bread	100% whole-wheat bread	Baguettes
Barley kernel bread	Corn tortillas, wheat tortillas	English muffins
Rye kernel bread	Cracked-wheat kernel bread	Gluten-free white bread
Whole-wheat kernel bread	Hearty 7-grain bread	Hamburger buns
	Oat bran bread	Middle Eastern flatbread
	Pita bread	Rice bread
	Whole-wheat spelt bread	Wheat bagels
	Whole-grain pumpernickel	White bread

Breakfast Cereals

Low GI: 55 or less (good choice)	Moderate GI: 56–69	High GI: 70 or higher (avoid/limit)
All-Bran	Bran Chex	Bran Flakes
Fiber One	Kashi Go LEAN	Cheerios
Oat bran	Kashi Good Friends	Chex (rice or corn)
Rice bran	Kellogg's Mini-Wheats	Corn Bran
	Nutrigrain	Cornflakes
	Oatmeal (slow cook)	Corn Pops
	Raisin Bran	Cream of Wheat
	Toasted muesli	Granola
	Whole-wheat Special K	Grape-Nuts
		Oatmeal (instant)
		Puffed Wheat
		Rice Krispies
		Sugary cereals
		Shredded Wheat
		Total

Cereal Grains (cooked)

Low GI: 55 or less (good choice)	Moderate GI: 56–69	High GI: 70 or higher (avoid/limit)
Barley, pearled or cracked Brown rice Buckwheat Buckwheat groats Bulgur (cracked wheat) Quinoa Whole kernel rye Whole kernel wheat	Basmati rice Cornmeal Couscous Long grain rice (boiled 10 minutes) Rolled barley	Jasmine white rice Millet Parboiled rice Quick-cooking rice White rice

Dairy

Low GI: 55 or less (good choice)	Moderate GI: 56–69	High GI: 70 or higher (avoid/limit)
Organic plain low-fat or nonfat yogurt Organic milk	Low-fat or nonfat fruit yogurt	Frozen yogurt Tofu frozen dessert

Fruit

Low GI: 55 or less (good choice)	Moderate GI: 56–69	High GI: 70 or higher (avoid/limit)
Apple	Apple juice (unsweetened)	Canned fruits in syrup
Berries, frozen or fresh	Banana	Dates
Cherries	Cantaloupe	Fruit cocktails
Grapes	Carrot juice (fresh)	Fruit juices with added sugar
Grapefruit	Grapefruit juice (unsweetened)	Raisins
Orange	Kiwi	Watermelon
Peach	Mango	
Pear	Orange juice (unsweetened)	
Plum	Papaya	
	Pineapple	

Legumes

Low GI: 55 or less (good choice)	Moderate GI: 56–69	High GI: 70 or higher (avoid/limit)
Baby lima beans Black beans Black-eyed peas Chickpeas (garbanzo beans) Kidney beans Lentils Mung beans Pinto beans Romano beans Soy beans Split peas	Navy beans	Baked beans (canned) Broad beans Navy beans (pressure cooked >25 minutes)

Pasta

Low GI: 55 or less (good choice)	Moderate GI: 56–69	High GI: 70 or higher (avoid/limit)
Fettuccini, egg-enriched Lentil pasta Quinoa pasta Spaghetti (whole wheat) Spinach pasta	Capellini Macaroni (boiled 5 min) Rice noodles, dried Spaghetti (cooked al dente) Udon noodles	Gnocchi Spaghetti (boiled more than 20 minutes)

Vegetables

Low GI: 55 or less (good choice)	Moderate GI: 56–69	High GI: 70 or higher (avoid/ limit)
Asparagus	Beets	Instant potatoes
Broccoli	Green peas	Russet potato
Brussels sprouts	Sweet corn	New potato
Bok choy	Sweet potato	French fries
Cabbage	Yam	Winter squash
Carrots		Pumpkin
Cauliflower		
Eggplant		
Dark leafy greens		
Romaine lettuce		
Mushrooms		
Green peas		
Peppers		
Snow peas		
Spinach		
Summer squash		
Tomatoes		
Tomato juice		
Zucchini		

Snacks

Low GI: 55 or less (good choice)	Moderate GI: 56–69	High GI: 70 or higher (avoid/limit)
Nuts and seeds, including almonds, peanuts, and walnuts	Breton wheat crackers Protein bars Rye crispbread crackers	Breakfast cereal bars Candy Chocolate (especially sweetened milk chocolate) Cookies Corn chips Jelly beans Melba toast Muesli bars Popcorn Potato chips Pretzels Rice cakes Saltines Sports drinks (Gatorade)

Sweeteners

Low GI: 55 or less (good choice)	Moderate GI: 56–69	High GI: 70 or higher (avoid/limit)
Coconut crystals	Glucose Honey Sucrose	Maltose

APPENDIX E

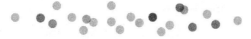

The Calming Power of Mantra

The mantra is a tool for calming the mind. *Mantra* stands for a word or short phrase that you repeat silently to yourself. The mantra works fast; it has the power to calm and steady your mind, stop you from reacting too quickly, and stop panic and fear. This skill is thousands of years old. St. Francis of Assisi used to repeat, "My God and my all."

Once you choose your mantra, silently repeat it as often as possible throughout the day. I use my mantra all day long, when I need it and when I don't (except when I need my full attention on a project). Don't wait until you feel stressed to use it. By using your mantra during nonstressful times, it will be available for you when you need it.

When to Use Mantra Repetition

You can use your mantra throughout the day, such as in the following situations:

- Standing in lines
- Being questioned by an authority such as a customs agent
- While on hold on the telephone
- When under stress while driving
- During arguments or disagreements with others
- While waiting for the elevator
- Prior to a job interview

- Before speaking in public
- Before answering the phone
- When sick and dealing with pain, illness, or surgery
- Before meals, to eat slowly
- Before sleep to help with insomnia

Use your mantra during daily tasks (mechanical ones that don't require your full attention). It is nice to play your mantra as background music in your home if it is available. (Check out iTunes and type in your mantra; it may have been put to music.)

- Washing dishes, sweeping, vacuuming, dusting
- Gardening and watering plants
- Dressing, bathing, showering
- While exercising—any repeated exercise where no special equipment is needed.

Use your mantra to calm unwanted emotions, such as:

- Ruminating and intrusive thoughts
- Fear
- Frustration
- Anger or rage
- Greed, resentment
- Worry
- Anxiety

Use your mantra to quiet yourself and bring attention into the present moment.

Mantra Repetition for Rapid Relaxation

Many of the following mantras were used by Jill Bormann in her PTSD research.

Mantra (pronunciation)	Description
Om mani padme hum (Ohm Mah-nee Pahd-may Hume)	An invocation to the jewel (Self) in the lotus of the heart
Namo Butsaya (Nah-mo Boot-sie-yah)	I bow to the Buddha
My God and my All	St. Francis of Assisi's mantra
Maranatha (Mar-ah-nah-tha)	Lord of the Heart [Aramaic]
Kyrie eleison (Kir-ee-ay Ee-lay-ee-sone)	Lord, have mercy
Jesus, Jesus or Lord Jesus Christ	Son of God
Hail Mary, full of grace; the Lord is with you [me]	Catholic rosary
Lord Jesus Christ, Son of God, have mercy on us [me]	Jesus prayer
Rama (Rah-mah)	Eternal joy within (Gandhi's mantra)
Om namah shivaya (Ohm Nah-mah Shee-vah-yah)	An invocation to beauty and fearlessness
Om prema (Ohm Pray-Mah)	A call for universal love
Om shanti (Ohm Shawn-tee)	An invocation to eternal peace
So hum (So Hum)	I am that Self within
Barukh atah Adonai (Bah-rookh At-tah Ah-doh-nigh)	Blessed art Thou, King of the Universe
Ribono shel olam (Ree-boh-no Shel O-lahm)	Master of the Universe
Shalom (Shah-lohm)	Peace, wellness
Sheheena (Sha-khee-nah)	Feminine aspect of God
Allah (Ah-lah)	The Supreme Being

Allahu akbar (Ah-lah-oo Ah-bahr)	God is greatest
Bismallah ir-rahman ir-rahim (Beese-mah-lah Ir-rah-mun Ir-rah-heem)	In the name of Allah, the merciful, the compassionate
Wakan Tanka (Wah-Kah Tahn-Kah)	Great Spirit
Om Namo Narayani	I surrender to the Divine

• ● •

APPENDIX F

Homeopathy First-Aid Kit

Homeopathy can be used in acute situations for self-limiting complaints such as those following an injury, or for more chronic conditions such as depression. Remedies to treat acute infection are used more frequently and are of lower potency. The usual dose is 3 to 5 pellets or tablets in a single dose on or under the tongue. Your health-care provider can guide you on the dosing that is best for you.

When taking a homeopathic remedy made of pellets, do not touch the remedy with your hands. Avoid consuming coffee or mints, and have a clean mouth. Take your remedy about 30 minutes before or after eating. Certain remedies, like Arnica, come in a cream form and can be applied topically.

Arnica (mountain daisy)

- The first remedy to give for accidents of any type
- Always the first remedy for head injury
- Use before and after surgery to support healing
- Use to help reduce pain and swelling
- Use topically for bruises on unbroken skin

Hypericum (St. John's wort)

- Great remedy for nerve injuries, especially fingers and toes
- Considered the "arnica" of the spinal column
- Use for surgical incisions
- Use for nerve pain

Ruta graveolens (rue, bitterwort)

- Best for ligamentous and tendon injuries
- Used for sprains after Arnica

Symphytum (Symphytum officinale)

- Excellent for fractures
- Especially good for nonunion fractures

Belladonna (deadly nightshade)

- Classic remedy for strep throat
- Use when intense heat, redness, throbbing and swelling
- Use for fever
- Use for earache

Oscillococcinum (heart and lung of duck)

- Use to treat and prevent influenza: 1 capful, three times daily
- Dose 1 capful daily if exposed to flu in the family
- Dose 1 capful weekly during flu season to prevent

Ipecac (ipecac root)

- Use for persistent nausea and vomiting
- Helpful for morning sickness
- Use for gastroenteritis, food poisoning (after using Nux vomica)

Nux vomica (poison nut)

- A remedy for those who are overindulgent or excessive
- For quick, active, nervous and irritable Type A personalities

- For people who are oversensitive to noise and who crave stimulants, drugs, and alcohol
- Use for hangovers and toxic exposures

Chamomilla (German chamomile)

- Use when your chief symptoms are emotional
- Used frequently in restless, irritable, whining, colicky children
- Commonly used for teething pain and earaches

Rhus tox (poison oak)

- Use for skin rashes, especially poison ivy
- Use for burns, such as sunburn
- Use for strained joints or tendons

Ledum (marsh tea)

- Use for puncture wounds produced by bites or sharp instruments
- Excellent for insect bites
- Helpful before getting injections

Calendula (pot marigold)

- Use topically for open cuts
- Use on infected skin
- Use for irritating rashes, including diaper rash

• ● •

BIBLIOGRAPHY

Action for Health in Diabetes (Look AHEAD) Study Group. Association of weight loss main-tenance and weight regain on 4-year changes in CVD risk factors: the Action for Health in Diabetes (Look AHEAD) Clinical Trial. *Diabetes Care*. 2016 Aug;39(8):1345–55.

Anderson JW, Liu C, Kryscio RJ. Blood pressure response to transcendental meditation: a meta-analysis. *Am J Hypertens*. 2008 Mar;21(3):310–6.

Apaydin EA, Maher AR, Shanman R et al. A systematic review of St. John's wort for major depressive disorder. *Syst Rev*. 2016 Sep 2;5(1):148.

Appel LJ, Moore TJ, Obarzanek E et al. A clinical trial of the effects of dietary patterns on blood pressure. DASH Collaborative Research Group. *N Engl J Med*. 1997;336(16):1117–24.

Ariyo AA, Haan M, Tangen CM et al. Depressive symptoms and risks of coronary heart disease and mortality in elderly Americans. Cardiovascular Health Study Collaborative Research Group. *Circulation*. 2000 Oct 10;102(15):1773–9.

Bernardi L. Effect of rosary prayer and yoga mantras on autonomic cardiovascular rhythms: comparative study. *BMJ* 2001;323:1446–49 (22–29 Dec).

Bormann JE. Frequent, silent mantram repetition: a Jacuzzi for the mind. *Top Emerg Med*. 2005 Apr/Jun;27(2):163–66.

Budoff MJ, Takasu J, Flores FR et al. Inhibiting progression of coronary calcification using aged garlic extract in patients receiving statin therapy: a preliminary study. *Prev Med*. 2004 Nov;39(5):985–91.

Caminiti G, Volterrani M, Marazzi G et al. Tai chi enhances the effects of endurance train-ing in the rehabilitation of elderly patients with chronic heart failure. *Rehabil Res Pract*. 2011;2011:761958. doi: 10.1155/2011/761958. Epub 2010 Sep 13.

Campello E, Spiezia L, Simioni P. Diagnosis and management of factor V Leiden. *Expert Rev Hematol*. 2016 Oct 31:1–11.

Carwile JL, Ye X, Zhou X et al. Canned soup consumption and urinary bisphenol A: a ran-domized crossover trial. *JAMA*. 2011 Nov 23;306(20):2218–20.

Cohen S, Doyle WJ, Skoner DP et al. Social ties and susceptibility to the common cold. *JAMA* 1997 Jun 25;277(24):1940–44.

Creswell JD, Lam S, Stanton AL et al. Does self-affirmation, cognitive processing, or discovery of meaning explain cancer-related health benefits of expressive writing? *Pers Soc Psychol Bull*. 2007 Feb;33(2):238–50.

De Lorgeril M. Mediterranean diet and cardiovascular disease: historical perspective and latest evidence. *Curr Atheroscler Rep*. 2013 Dec;15(12):370.

De Vogli R, Chandola T, Marmot MG. Negative aspects of close relationships and heart dis-ease. *Arch Intern Med*. 2007;167:1951–57.

Demeyer D, Mertens B, De Smet S et al. Mechanisms linking colorectal cancer to the con-sumption of (processed) red meat: a review. *Crit Rev Food Sci Nutr*. 2016 Dec 9;56(16):2747–66.

Deng G, Hou BL, Holodny AI et al. Functional magnetic resonance imaging (fMRI) changes and saliva production associated with acupuncture at LI-2 acupuncture point: a randomized controlled study. *BMC Complement Altern Med*. 2008 Jul 7;8:37.

Derikx LA, Dieleman LA, Hoentjen F. Probiotics and prebiotics in ulcerative colitis. *Best Pract Res Clin Gastroenterol*. 2016 Feb;30(1):55–71.

Drago F, Ciccarese G, Parodi A. Nicotinamide for skin-cancer chemoprevention. *N Engl J Med.* 2016 Feb 25;374(8):789–90. doi: 10.1056/NEJMc1514791#SA2.

Egolf B, Lasker J, Wolf S et al. The Roseto effect: a 50-year comparison of mortality rates. *Am J Public Health.* 1992 Aug;82(8):1089–92.

Emmett PM, Jones LR, Golding J. Pregnancy diet and associated outcomes in the Avon Longitudinal Study of Parents and Children. *Nutr Rev.* 2015 Oct;73 Suppl 3:154–74.

Environmental News Service. EPA must rewrite plastic factories' emission standards. 2005 April 25. Online: http://www.ens-newswire.com/ens/apr2005/2005-04-25-09.asp#anchor2 (21 October 2009).

EPA's 2008 report on the environment, https://cfpub.epa.gov/ncea/risk/recordisplay.cfm?deid=190806.

Epel ES, Blackburn EH, Lin J. Accelerated telomere shortening in response to life stress. *PNAS.* 101(49):17312–15.

Feifel D, Pappas K. Treating clinical depression with repetitive deep transcranial magnetic stimulation using the brainsway H1-coil. *J Vis Exp.* 2016 Oct 4;(116).

Feola A, Ricci S, Kouidhi S et al. Multifaceted breast cancer: the molecular connection with obesity. *J Cell Physiol.* 2017 Jan;232(1):69–77. doi: 10.1002/jcp.25475. Epub 2016 Jul 21.

Ferrara LA, Raimondi AS, d'Episcopo L. Olive oil and reduced need for antihypertensive medications. *Arch Intern Med.* 2000 Mar 27;160(6):837–42.

Fournier JC, DeRubeis RJ, Hollon SD et al. Antidepressant drug effects and depression severity: a patient-level meta-analysis. *JAMA.* 2010 Jan 6;303(1):47–53.

Gibson CM, Pride YB, Hochberg CP et al. Effect of intensive statin therapy on clinical outcomes among patients undergoing percutaneous coronary intervention for acute coronary syndrome. PCI-PROVE IT: A PROVE IT-TIMI 22 (Pravastatin or Atorvastatin Evaluation and Infection Therapy-Thrombolysis in Myocardial Infarction 22) Substudy. *J Am Coll Cardiol.* 2009 Dec 8;54(24):2290–5.

Girotra M, Garg S, Anand R et al. Fecal microbiota transplantation for recurrent Clostridium difficile infection in the elderly: long-term outcomes and microbiota changes. *Dig Dis Sci.* 2016 Oct;61(10):3007–15. doi: 10.1007/s10620-016-4229-8. Epub 2016 Jul 22.

Hojat M, Louis DZ, Markham FW et al. Physicians' empathy and clinical outcomes for diabetic patients. *Acad Med.* 2011 Mar;86(3):359–64.

Innes KE, Selfe TK, Khalsa DS et al. Stress, mood, sleep, and quality of life in adults with early memory loss: a pilot randomized controlled trial. *J Alzheimers Dis.* 2016 Apr 8;52(4):1277–98.

IPCC. Summary for Policymakers. In: Edenhofer O, Pichs-Madruga R, Sokona Y et al. Climate Change 2014, Mitigation of Climate Change Contribution of Working Group III to the Fifth Assessment Report of the Intergovernmental Panel on Climate Change. Cambridge, United Kingdom and New York, NY: Cambridge University Press, 2014.

Irwin MR, Olmstead R, Carroll JE. Sleep disturbance, sleep duration, and inflammation: a systematic review and meta-analysis of cohort studies and experimental sleep deprivation. *Biol Psychiatry.* 2016 Jul 1;80(1):40–52. doi: 10.1016/j.biopsych.2015.05.014. Epub 2015 Jun 1.

Jain S, McMahon GF, Hasen P et al. Healing touch with guided imagery for PTSD in returning active duty military: a randomized controlled trial. *Mil Med.* 2012 Sep;177(9):1015–21.

Ji S, Wang F, Chen Y et al. Developmental changes in the level of free and conjugated sialic acids, Neu5Ac, Neu5Gc and KDN in different organs of pig: a LC-MS/MS quantitative analyses. *Glycoconj J.* 2016 Sep 9. [Epub ahead of print.]

Johnston BC, Goldenberg JZ, Parkin PC. Probiotics and the prevention of antibiotic-associated diarrhea in infants and children. *JAMA.* 2016 Oct 11;316(14):1484–5.

Kastelein JJ, Maki KC, Susekov A et al. Omega-3 free fatty acids for the treatment of severe hypertriglyceridemia: the EpanoVa fOr Lowering Very high triglyceridEs (EVOLVE) trial. *J Clin Lipidol.* 2014 Jan-Feb;8(1):94–106. doi: 10.1016/j.jacl.2013.10.003. Epub 2013 Oct 14.

Kirsch I, Deacon BJ, Huedo-Medina TB et al. Initial severity and antidepressant benefits: a meta-analysis of data submitted to the Food and Drug Administration. *PLoS Med.* 2008

Feb;5(2):e45. doi: 10.1371/journal.pmed.0050045.

Kleijnen J, Knipschild P, ter Riet G. Clinical trials of homoeopathy. *BMJ* 1991 Feb 9;302(6772):316–23.

Knoops KT, de Groot LC, Kromhout D et al. Mediterranean diet, lifestyle factors, and 10-year mortality in elderly European men and women: the HALE project. *JAMA.* 2004 Sep 22;292(12):1433–9.

Kumar M, Kissoon-Singh V, Leon Coria A et al. The probiotic mixture VSL#3 reduces colonic inflammation and improves intestinal barrier function in Muc2 mucin deficient mice. *Am J Physiol Gastrointest Liver Physiol.* 2016 Nov 17. doi: 10.1152/ajpgi.00298.2016.

Lam RW, Levitt AJ, Levitan RD et al. The Can-SAD study: a randomized controlled trial of the effectiveness of light therapy and fluoxetine in patients with winter seasonal affective disorder. *Am J Psychiatry.* 2006 May;163(5):805–12.

Legrand FD, Neff EM. Efficacy of exercise as an adjunct treatment for clinically depressed inpatients during the initial stages of antidepressant pharmacotherapy: an open randomized controlled trial. *J Affect Disord.* 2016 Feb;191:139–44. doi: 10.1016/j.jad.2015.11.047. Epub 2015 Nov 30.

Lemoine P, Wade AG, Katz A et al. Efficacy and safety of prolonged-release melatonin for insomnia in middle-aged and elderly patients with hypertension: a combined analysis of controlled clinical trials. *Integr Blood Press Control.* 2012;5:9–17. Epub 2012 Jan 25.

Lengacher CA, Reich RR, Kip KE et al. Influence of mindfulness-based stress reduction (MBSR) on telomerase activity in women with breast cancer (BC). *Biol Res Nurs.* 2014 Oct;16(4):438–47.

Leor J, Poole WK, Kloner RA. Sudden cardiac death triggered by an earthquake. *N Engl J Med.* 1996;334:413–19.

Lerner-Ellis J, Khalouei S, Sopik V et al. Genetic risk assessment and prevention: the role of genetic testing panels in breast cancer. *Expert Rev Anticancer Ther.* 2015;15(11):1315–26.

Li Y, Jiang L, Jia Z et al. A meta-analysis of red yeast rice: an effective and relatively safe alternative approach for dyslipidemia. *PLoS One.* 2014 Jun 4;9(6): 2014.

MacKay D, Hathcock J, Guarneri E. Niacin: chemical forms, bioavailability, and health effects. *Nutr Rev.* 2012 Jun;70(6):357–66. doi: 10.1111/j.1753-4887.2012.00479.x.

Marucha PT, Kiecolt-Glaser J, Favagehi M. Mucosal wound healing is impaired by examination stress. *Psychosomatic Medicine.* 1998;60(3):362–65.

McConnel CS, Stenkamp-Strahm CM, Rao S et al. Antimicrobial resistance profiles in Escherichia coli O157 isolates from northern Colorado dairies. *J Food Prot.* 2016 Mar;79(3):484–7.

Millennium Ecosystem Assessment www.millenniumassessment.org/en/index.html.

Miller PE, Van Elswyk M, Alexander DD. Long-chain omega-3 fatty acids eicosapentaenoic acid and docosahexaenoic acid and blood pressure: a meta-analysis of randomized controlled trials. *Am J Hypertens.* 2014 Jul;27(7):885–96. doi: 10.1093/ajh/hpu024. Epub 2014 Mar 6.

Momose Y, Maeda-Yamamoto M, Nabetani H. Systematic review of green tea epigallocatechin gallate in reducing low-density lipoprotein cholesterol levels of humans. *Int J Food Sci Nutr.* 2016 Sep;67(6):606–13. doi: 10.1080/09637486.2016.1196655. Epub 2016 Jun 20.

Monaco P, Quattrocchi F. [Study of the antidepressive effects of a biological transmethylating agent (S-adenosyl-methione or SAM).] *Riv Neurol.* 1979 Nov-Dec;49(6):417–39.

Mostofsky E, Penner EA, Mittleman MA. Outbursts of anger as a trigger of acute cardiovascular events: a systematic review and meta-analysis. *Eur Heart J.* 2014 Jun 1;35(21):1404–10. doi: 10.1093/eurheartj/ehu033. Epub 2014 Mar 3.

Mueller PS, Plevak DJ, Rummans TA. Religious involvement, spirituality, and medicine: implications for clinical practice. *Mayo Clin Proc.* 2001 Dec;76(12):1225–35.

Murabito JM. Women and cardiovascular disease: contributions from the Framingham Heart Study. *J Am Med Womens Assoc.* 1995 Mar-Apr;50(2):35–9, 55.

NIH Consensus Conference. Acupuncture. *JAMA.* 1998 Nov 4;280(17):1518–24.

Ornish D, Lin J, Chan JM et al. Effect of comprehensive lifestyle changes on telomerase activity and telomere length in men with biopsy-proven low-risk prostate cancer: 5-year follow-up of a descriptive pilot study. *Lancet Oncol.* 2013 Oct;14(11):1112–20.

Pan L, Yan J, Guo Y et al. Effects of tai chi training on exercise capacity and quality of life in patients with chronic heart failure: a meta-analysis. *Eur J Heart Fail.* 2013 Mar;15(3):316–23.

Parker GB, Brotchie H, Graham RK. Vitamin D and depression. *J Affect Disord.* 2016 Oct 11;208:56–61.

Petridou ET, Kousoulis AA, Michelakos T et al. Folate and B12 serum levels in association with depression in the aged: a systematic review and meta-analysis. *Aging Ment Health.* 2016 Sep;20(9):965–73. doi: 10.1080/13607863.2015.1049115. Epub 2015 Jun 8.

Ras RT, Geleijnse JM, Trautwein EA. LDL-cholesterol-lowering effect of plant sterols and stanols across different dose ranges: a meta-analysis of randomised controlled studies. *Br J Nutr.* 2014 Jul 28;112(2):214–9. doi: 10.1017/S0007114514000750. Epub 2014 Apr 29.

Reynolds T. Contamination of PC-SPES remains a mystery. *J Natl Cancer Inst.* 2002 Sep 4;94(17):1266–8.

Robine JM, Cheung SL, Le Roy S et al. Death toll exceeded 70,000 in Europe during the summer of 2003. *C R Biol.* 2008;331(2):171–8.

Rochester JR. Bisphenol A and human health: a review of the literature. *Reprod Toxicol.* 2013 Dec;42:132–55.

S. 784 — 103rd Congress: Dietary Supplement Health and Education Act of 1994. Public Law 103-417.

Schneider RH, Grim CE, Rainforth MV. Stress reduction in the secondary prevention of cardiovascular disease: randomized, controlled trial of transcendental meditation and health education in blacks. *Circ Cardiovasc Qual Outcomes.* 2012 Nov;5(6):750–8. Epub 2012 Nov 13.

Sihvonen R, Paavola M, Malmivaara A et al.; Finnish Degenerative Meniscal Lesion Study (FIDELITY) Group. Arthroscopic partial meniscectomy versus sham surgery for a degenerative meniscal tear. *N Engl J Med.* 2013 Dec 26;369(26):2515–24.

Sirtori CR, Arnoldi A, Cicero AF. Nutraceuticals for blood pressure control. *Ann Med.* 2015;47(6):447–56.

Steinberg JS, Arshad A, Kowalski M et al. Increased incidence of life-threatening ventricular arrhythmias in implantable defibrillator patients after the World Trade Center attack. *J Am Coll Cardiol.* 2004;44(6):1261–64.

Stokstad E. Toxicology. Salmon survey stokes debate about farmed fish. *Science.* 2004 Jan 9;303(5655):154–5.

Strassner C, Cavoski I, Di Cagno R et al. How the organic food system supports sustainable diets and translates these into practice. *Front Nutr.* 2015 Jun 29;2:19. doi: 10.3389/fnut.2015.00019. eCollection 2015.

Surampudi P, Enkhmaa B, Anuurad E et al. Lipid lowering with soluble dietary fiber. *Curr Atheroscler Rep.* 2016 Dec;18(12):75.

Sutton R. Chromium-6 in U.S. Tap Water, 2010, www.ewg.org/chromium6-in-tap-water.

Tibbits D, Ellis G, Piramelli C et al. Hypertension reduction through forgiveness training. J Pastoral Care Counsel. 2006 Spring-Summer;60(1-2):27–34.

Toxic substances control act, 15 U.S.C. §2601 et seq. (1976).

Turner JM, Spatz ES. Nutritional supplements for the treatment of hypertension: a practical guide for clinicians. Curr Cardiol Rep. 2016 Dec;18(12):126.

Tusek DL, Church JM, Strong SA et al. Guided imagery: a significant advance in the care of patients undergoing elective colorectal surgery. Dis Colon Rectum. 1997 Feb;40(2):172–8.

U.S. Food & Drug Administration. Dietary Supplements Guidance Documents & Regulatory Information, 2007.

Van Niel C, Pachter LM, Wade R Jr et al. Adverse events in children: predictors of adult physical and mental conditions. J Dev Behav Pediatr. 2014 Oct;35(8):549–51.

WHO fact sheet on Antibiotic Resistance 2016, www.who.int/mediacentre/factsheets/fs194/en/.

WHO. Quantitative risk assessment of the effects of climate change on selected causes of death, 2030s and 2050s. Geneva: World Health Organization, 2014.

Wider B, Pittler MH, Thompson-Coon J et al. Artichoke leaf extract for treating hypercholesterolaemia. Cochrane Database Syst Rev. 2013 Mar 28;(3):CD003335. doi: 10.1002/14651858.CD003335.

Yu H, Li C, Yang J et al. Berberine is a potent agonist of peroxisome proliferator activate receptor alpha. Front Biosci (Landmark Ed). 2016 Jun 1;21:1052–60.

Zhang X, Li Y, Del Gobbo LC et al. Effects of magnesium supplementation on blood pressure: a meta-analysis of randomized double-blind placebo-controlled trials. Hypertension. 2016 Aug;68(2):324–33. Epub 2016 Jul 11.

ABOUT THE AUTHOR

Mimi Guarneri, M.D., FACC, is board certified in cardiology, internal medicine, nuclear cardiology, and holistic medicine. She is past president of the American Board of Integrative Holistic Medicine (ABIHM), founder and current president of the Academy of Integrative Health and Medicine (AIHM), and past president of the American Board of Integrative Holistic Medicine. Dr. Guarneri currently serves on the founding board of the American Board of Physician Specialties (ABPS) in Integrative Medicine and is a clinical associate professor at University of California, San Diego (UCSD).

After receiving her undergraduate degree in English literature from New York University, Dr. Guarneri earned medical degree from SUNY Medical Center in New York, where she graduated number one in her class. She served her internship and residency at Cornell Medical Center, where she later became chief medical resident. She served cardiology fellowships at both New York University Medical Center and Scripps Clinic. She is a fellow member of the American College of Cardiology, Alpha Omega Alpha Honor Medical Society, and the American Medical Women's Association.

Dr. Guarneri began her career at Scripps Clinic as an attending in interventional cardiology, where she placed thousands of coronary stents. Recognizing the need for a more comprehensive and more holistic approach to cardiovascular disease, she co-founded the Scripps Center for Integrative Medicine, where she pioneered state-of-the-art cardiac imaging technology and lifestyle change programs to aggressively diagnose, prevent and treat cardiovascular disease. She co-founded and is current medical director of Guarneri Integrative Health, Inc., at Pacific Pearl La Jolla in California, where she leads her team of experts in conventional, integrative, and natural medicine.

She is the author of *The Heart Speaks*, a poignant collection of stories from heart patients who have benefited from integrative medicine approaches. *The Heart Speaks* and Dr. Guarneri's clinical work have been featured on television at NBC's *Today* and PBS's *To the Contrary* and *Full Focus*. Her work also was featured in a two-part PBS documentary, *The New Medicine*.

Dr. Guarneri has been recognized for her national leadership in integrative medicine by the Bravewell Collaborative and has served as chair of the Bravewell Clinical Network for Integrative Medicine. In 2009, Dr. Guarneri was honored as the ARCS scientist of the year. In 2011, Dr. Guarneri was the winner of the Bravewell Leadership Award, which honors a physician leader who has made significant contributions to the transformation of the U.S. health-care system. In 2012, she received the Linus Pauling Functional Medicine Lifetime Achievement Award from the Institute for Functional Medicine and the Grace A. Goldsmith Award from the American College of Nutrition.

Websites: www.mimiguarnerimd.com,
www.miraglofoundation.org,
and www.facebook.com/PacificPearlLaJolla

We hope you enjoyed this Hay House book. If you'd like to receive our online catalog featuring additional information on Hay House books and products, or if you'd like to find out more about the Hay Foundation, please contact:

Hay House, Inc., P.O. Box 5100, Carlsbad, CA 92018-5100
(760) 431-7695 or (800) 654-5126
(760) 431-6948 (fax) or (800) 650-5115 (fax)
www.hayhouse.com® • www.hayfoundation.org

• • •

Published and distributed in Australia by: Hay House Australia Pty. Ltd.,
18/36 Ralph St., Alexandria NSW 2015 • *Phone:* 612-9669-4299
Fax: 612-9669-4144 • www.hayhouse.com.au

Published and distributed in the United Kingdom by: Hay House UK, Ltd.,
Astley House, 33 Notting Hill Gate, London W11 3JQ • *Phone:* 44-20-3675-2450
Fax: 44-20-3675-2451 • www.hayhouse.co.uk

Published and distributed in the Republic of South Africa by:
Hay House SA (Pty), Ltd., P.O. Box 990, Witkoppen 2068
info@hayhouse.co.za_ * www.hayhouse.co.za

Published in India by: Hay House Publishers India, Muskaan Complex,
Plot No. 3, B-2, Vasant Kunj, New Delhi 110 070 • *Phone:* 91-11-4176-1620
Fax: 91-11-4176-1630 • www.hayhouse.co.in

Distributed in Canada by: Raincoast Books, 2440 Viking Way, Richmond, B.C.
V6V 1N2 • *Phone:* 1-800-663-5714 • *Fax:* 1-800-565-3770 • www.raincoast.com

• • •

Take Your Soul on a Vacation

Visit www.HealYourLife.com® to regroup, recharge, and reconnect with your own magnificence.
Featuring blogs, mind-body-spirit news, and life-changing wisdom from Louise Hay and friends.

Visit www.HealYourLife.com today!

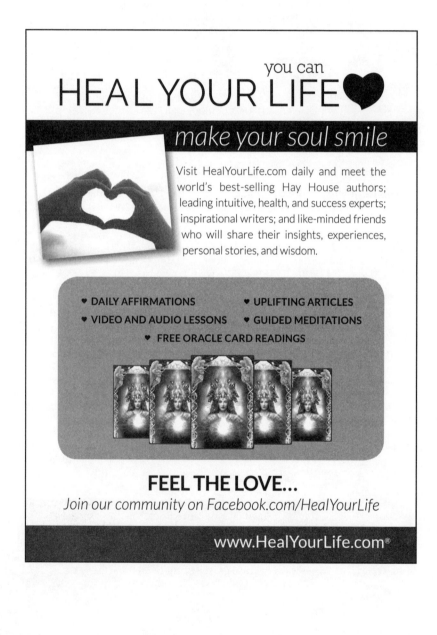